Rapid Medicines Management for Healthcare Professionals

T0176973

Rapid Medicines Management for Healthcare Professionals

Paul Deslandes BPharm, PhD, MRSB, CBiol, AFHEA
Senior Lecturer
Faculty of Life Sciences and Education
University of South Wales
Pontypridd, UK

Simon Young BPharm, PhD, MRPharmS, SFHEA
Academic Subject Manager and Head of Post Registration Provision
Faculty of Life Sciences and Education
University of South Wales
Pontypridd, UK

Ben Pitcher BSc, BN, FHEA
Senior Lecturer
Faculty of Life Sciences and Education
University of South Wales
Pontypridd, UK

WILEY Blackwell

Registered Office(s)
John Wiley & Sons, Inc., 111 River Street, Hoboken, NJ 07030, USA
John Wiley & Sons Ltd, The Atrium, Southern Gate, Chichester, West Sussex, PO19 8SQ, UK

Editorial Office
9600 Garsington Road, Oxford, OX4 2DQ, UK

For details of our global editorial offices, customer services, and more information about Wiley products visit us at www.wiley.com.

Wiley also publishes its books in a variety of electronic formats and by print-on-demand. Some content that appears in standard print versions of this book may not be available in other formats.

Library of Congress Cataloging-in-Publication Data

Names: Deslandes, Paul, author. | Young, Simon, 1971– author. | Pitcher, Ben, 1979– author.
Title: Rapid medicines management for healthcare professionals / Paul Deslandes, Simon Young, Ben Pitcher.
Description: Hoboken, NJ : John Wiley & Sons, Inc., 2020. | Includes bibliographical references and index.
Identifiers: LCCN 2019024487| ISBN 9781119397724 (paperback) | ISBN 9781119397755 (adobe pdf) | ISBN 9781119397885 (epub)
Subjects: | MESH: Drug Therapy–nursing | Drug Therapy–methods | Drug Prescriptions–nursing | Pharmacological Phenomena | Handbook
Classification: LCC RM301 | NLM WY 49 | DDC 615.1–dc23 LC record available at https://lccn.loc.gov/2019024487

Cover Design: Wiley
Cover Image: © Nipitphon Na Chiangmai/Getty Images

Set in 7.5/9.5pt, FrutigerLTStd by SPi Global, Pondicherry, India
Printed and bound in Singapore by Markono Print Media Pte Ltd

10 9 8 7 6 5 4 3 2 1

Contents

Section III   Therapeutics, 97

Section IV Practice Considerations, 263

Introduction

The use of medicines in the management of disease is becoming increasingly complex. Advances in medical technologies, and the increasing incidence of co-morbidity and poly-pharmacy associated with an ageing population, present significant challenges to all healthcare professionals. The increased emphasis on medicines management in existing roles, alongside the proliferation of advanced practice roles, adds to the need for proficiency in this area.

In line with the need for effective medicines management, there is a vast and ever-expanding volume of published literature and treatment guidelines to inform decision making. However, these resources may be presented in an inaccessible way, particularly for those less familiar with the subject. The aim of this book is to introduce students and healthcare professionals who may be less well versed in this area to some of the key principles of pharmacology and medicines management. This book is not intended to replace, but instead to sit alongside and add context to other standard reference sources (such as the *British National Formulary*). In addition, the book does not replace guidelines, protocols, and other evidence-based texts. Professional judgement and up-to-date knowledge should always be applied in making clinical decisions directly affecting the health and well-being of patients.

We have divided the book into four broad sections. Whilst the sections have been organised into a logical sequence, the book is not necessarily intended to be read in any particular order. Most chapters can be read as stand-alone entities to obtain information on a given subject or drug. The first section introduces the reader to some fundamental principles of pharmacology, as well as to the terminology/vocabulary that is used in later sections to describe the properties of different drugs. For example, the term 'antagonist' is explained in Chapter 6 and used in later chapters where the mechanism of action of a specific drug or drug group is described. The second section considers the ways in which drugs are administered and how their actions can be affected when they are used for specific patient groups. In addition, this section includes chapters on adverse drug reactions and the mechanisms resulting in drug interactions.

Section III describes the actions, therapeutic effects, and adverse effects of some specific drugs or drug groups that are commonly used in practice in the UK. Each chapter is intended to provide a summary of key points and not an exhaustive account. These chapters use a common template, which is explained in more detail in Chapter 32. At the end of Section III you will find some blank templates that you may wish to complete yourself for drugs that are relevant to your area of practice but are not included. The final section of the book includes some practical considerations for the management of medicines, such as public health perspectives, legal aspects, and evidence-based medicine.

We have also included a glossary to give you easy access to explanations of certain pharmacological concepts and terminology that did not necessarily warrant chapters to themselves.

During our time teaching medicines management and pharmacology to pre-registration and post-registration students, many of them have told us how daunting this subject can be. This book was written for those students and practitioners who, like the ones we have spoken to, wanted some additional support in this area. We hope you find it informative and helpful.

SECTION I

Underpinning Theory

1 Introduction to Pharmacodynamics

Pharmacodynamics is often described as 'what the drug does to the body'. It is the study of how the drug interacts with a particular body system, and how it affects this system to bring about a therapeutic effect. The pharmacodynamic properties of a drug can help us to predict what side effects, adverse effects, and drug interactions we might expect to see when a drug (or combination of drugs) is used in practice.

Sites of drug action

The site of drug action within the body can be broadly divided into receptors, enzymes, and transmembrane transporters and channels. Many drugs will have an effect at more than one site, one of which may be the intended target to mediate the therapeutic effect. However, the other could be a different site, or a similar site located in a different part of the body, and which mediates a completely different effect from that intended. This forms the basis for some of the side effects that patients may experience. Competition between two or more drugs for a particular target may result in an increased or decreased effect, and is the basis for pharmacodynamic drug interactions.

Receptors

Receptors are specific sites, typically located on cell membranes, which are bound to by the body's endogenous signalling molecules (such as hormones and neurotransmitters). When these signalling molecules bind to the receptor, they bring about or mediate an effect. Drugs have been discovered which, due to their chemical structure, will also bind to these receptors within the body. Once bound, the drug may mimic the effect of the endogenous signalling molecule and bring about a physiological response. Alternatively, it may have no effect and prevent the action of the endogenous signalling molecule, blocking the normal response. Examples include salbutamol (which mimics the effect of endogenous adrenaline) and atenolol (which blocks the effect of endogenous adrenaline), used in the treatment of asthma and hypertension, respectively.

Enzymes

Enzymes are proteins that catalyse (facilitate) chemical reactions occurring in the body through an interaction with molecules at specific parts of their structures. Some drugs are able to interact with the enzyme either at its binding site (or sometimes elsewhere on its structure) and can interrupt this action. As a result, the physiological process that is mediated by the enzyme will be prevented. This might include inhibition of the normal breakdown of a neurotransmitter, prolonging its effect (e.g. the inhibition of acetylcholine

Rapid Medicines Management for Healthcare Professionals, First Edition. Paul Deslandes, Simon Young and Ben Pitcher.
© 2020 John Wiley & Sons Ltd. Published 2020 by John Wiley & Sons Ltd.

metabolism by donepezil). Alternatively, it could be the inhibition of the formation of a clotting factor, resulting in impaired blood clotting and an anticoagulant effect (e.g. the factor Xa inhibitor rivaroxaban).

Transport proteins and channels

The movement of many molecules and ions across cell membranes is facilitated by transport proteins and channels. These membrane-spanning proteins allow water-soluble substances to move across the lipid membranes responsible for maintaining cellular homeostasis. Preventing or in some cases facilitating the movement of these substances with drugs can result in a therapeutic effect. An example is the calcium channel blocker group of drugs, which prevent the movement of calcium ions into (and within) nerve cells and muscle cells, and which are used in the treatment of angina and hypertension.

Other sites of drug action

In addition to the above, drugs may also mediate their therapeutic effects through other actions within the body. Monoclonal antibody based therapies (such as adalimumab) bind to specific inflammatory proteins to prevent them from exerting their normal physiological effect. Osmotic laxatives (such as lactulose), maintain water in the colon by increasing the osmolarity when they are present in the gastrointestinal tract. Replacement therapies (such as fluids, electrolytes, and oxygen) are sometimes considered a separate group of medicines and could be considered less pharmacologically active in this regard. However, the molecule that is being replaced may have an action at one of the pharmacological sites of action mentioned above (examples include levothyroxine or insulin).

2 Synaptic Transmission

Many physiological processes occurring within the body are regulated by the nerve cells of the autonomic nervous system, or through the action of other neuronal pathways. Conduction of a signal or message (action potential) through an individual nerve cell utilises the properties of the neuronal membrane and its ability to conduct an electrical impulse. However, the arrangement of neurons in the autonomic nervous system results in junctions (synapses) between nerve cells or between nerve cells and their target tissue. These synapses (or 'synaptic clefts') are spaces through which the electrical conduction of an action potential cannot be transmitted. Consequently, an alternative means of conducting the signal from one cell to another must be used.

Synaptic transmission forms the basis through which signals are conducted from one nerve cell to another or from a nerve cell to its target tissue. The mechanism through which this is achieved is via a chemical signalling molecule. The chemical signalling molecule that allows transfer of a signal across the synapse is termed a neurotransmitter. The cell from which the neurotransmitter is released is termed 'presynaptic' and the second cell that receives the signal from the neurotransmitter is termed 'postsynaptic'.

The process through which a presynaptic neuron utilises a neurotransmitter to transmit a signal can be divided into five steps:

- neurotransmitter synthesis and storage
- neurotransmitter release
- receptor interaction
- neurotransmitter reuptake
- neurotransmitter metabolism.

Each of these steps provides a potential target for drug action and, as such, a way in which to manipulate physiological processes and treat symptoms of disease.

Neurotransmitter synthesis and storage

There are a number of different neurotransmitters in the body, each with their own chemical structure. Before a neurotransmitter can be released from the presynaptic neuron and exert an effect, it must first be synthesised. This process is typically facilitated by enzymes located in the presynaptic neuron, which convert a precursor chemical into the active neurotransmitter. Once synthesised, the neurotransmitter is typically stored in the presynaptic neuron (in a structure known as a vesicle) prior to its release in response to an action potential.

Medicines may promote the synthesis of neurotransmitters by providing additional amounts of the precursor chemical to the presynaptic neuron. Once converted to the neurotransmitter, there is a larger amount of neurotransmitter available to exert an effect. Examples of medicines that utilise this mechanism include levodopa (a precursor for the neurotransmitter dopamine), which is used in the management of Parkinson's disease.

Rapid Medicines Management for Healthcare Professionals, First Edition. Paul Deslandes, Simon Young and Ben Pitcher.
© 2020 John Wiley & Sons Ltd. Published 2020 by John Wiley & Sons Ltd.

Medicines may also interfere with the storage of neurotransmitters in vesicles. The medicine tetrabenazine reduces the transfer of the neurotransmitter dopamine into its storage vesicles, resulting in depletion of the neurotransmitter and a reduced effect. This forms the basis for the treatment of certain movement disorders associated with long-term antipsychotic use and symptoms of Huntington's disease.

Neurotransmitter release

Neurotransmitter release occurs in response to an action potential and typically involves the movement of calcium ions in the presynaptic neuron. Medicines inhibiting the influx of calcium into the neuron have the potential to reduce the release of a neurotransmitter, thereby reducing its effect. An example of this in practice is the opioid group of medicines used in the management of pain. Alternatively, neurotransmitter release may occur independently of the action of calcium. Drugs such as amfetamine can displace the neurotransmitter from its storage vesicle and into the synapse, resulting in a stimulant effect.

Receptor interaction

Once released from the presynaptic neuron, the neurotransmitter is able to exert an effect. This is typically achieved through an interaction with a receptor site located on a neuronal membrane or target tissue. There is a vast diversity of receptor types in the body, each able to interact with a specific neurotransmitter and mediate a physiological effect. Each neurotransmitter typically has more than one receptor group or subtype through which its effects are mediated. For example, there are seven groups of receptor for the neurotransmitter serotonin, most with a number of subtypes, resulting in more than ten individual receptor types for that neurotransmitter.

Both the neurotransmitter and the type of receptor with which it interacts will determine the resulting physiological effect. Some receptors have a stimulatory effect on the cell on which they are located, whilst others inhibit the activity of that cell. As a result, some neurotransmitters may have either stimulatory or inhibitory actions depending on the type of receptor with which they interact. For example, noradrenaline can cause vasodilatation through an action at one of its receptor subtypes, but vasoconstriction through a different receptor subtype.

A number of drugs exert their therapeutic effects through interactions with neurotransmitter receptors. Drugs may mimic the action of the body's own (endogenous) neurotransmitter and stimulate a receptor, enhancing a physiological effect (e.g. morphine, which stimulates opioid receptors, resulting in analgesia). Conversely, drugs may block receptors, preventing the endogenous neurotransmitter from binding and reducing the normal physiological effect (e.g. haloperidol, which blocks dopamine receptors and is used in the treatment of psychosis).

Neurotransmitter reuptake

In order to prevent continued stimulation of a receptor (and therefore stimulation of the tissue or organ on which it is located), which could be potentially harmful, the body has a mechanism for removing the neurotransmitter from the synaptic cleft. The cell membrane of the presynaptic neuron has a number of transport proteins (sometimes known as re-uptake transporters), which bind to the neurotransmitter and return it to the presynaptic neuron.

Certain drugs can inhibit reuptake transporter proteins, and in doing so enhance or prolong the effect of the neurotransmitter. By reducing re-uptake, the availability of the neurotransmitter in the synapse is increased, thereby increasing its ability to bind to receptors and exert an effect. Examples of drugs inhibiting serotonin reuptake include the antidepressants citalopram and fluoxetine (termed selective serotonin reuptake inhibitors).

Neurotransmitter metabolism

In addition to re-uptake, the effect of the neurotransmitter can also be terminated through the action of specific enzymes. Enzymes metabolise the neurotransmitter, altering its chemical structure and therefore preventing it from exerting an effect at its receptor site. Enzymatic degradation can take place in the synaptic cleft or in the presynaptic neuron following re-uptake.

Drugs may interact with the metabolic enzymes, inhibiting their action. This results in reduced degradation of the neurotransmitter, enhancing its effect. Drugs acting through this mechanism include donepezil (which reversibly inhibits the acetylcholinesterase enzyme responsible for metabolising acetylcholine), which is used in the treatment of dementia. Inhibition of the acetylcholinesterase enzyme also forms the basis of the mechanism of action of organophosphorus pesticides and the nerve agent sarin, which can result in poisoning following human exposure.

3   Neurotransmitters I

Neurotransmitters are signalling molecules released from neurons. They are released in small amounts with the intention of travelling the small distance from one neuron to another, or from a neuron onto a specific target organ or tissue. This is different to a hormone, which is released into the bloodstream and dispersed throughout the whole body. The difference between a hormone and a neurotransmitter is defined by how it is used by the body rather than anything inherent to its nature. For example, both adrenaline and noradrenaline can be released from the adrenal gland as hormones and can also be released from neurons as neurotransmitters.

Neurotransmitters are invariably agonists, eliciting a positive response when binding to their respective receptors. However, this response may have an inhibitory effect on the associated tissue or organ. For example, acetylcholine acts as an agonist on receptors on the heart, but the effect is to slow the heart down.

Autonomic nervous system

The autonomic nervous system (ANS) is an integral part of the body's homeostatic control system, regulating physiological factors such as blood pressure, pulse rate, vasoconstriction, bronchodilation, digestive function, and salivary secretions. As such, by stimulating or blocking the action of the associated neurotransmitters it is possible to exert control over this wide variety of processes. The ANS can be divided into the sympathetic and parasympathetic nervous systems, each with its own neurotransmitters and receptors.

Noradrenaline

Noradrenaline is described as a catecholamine, which describes a feature of its molecular structure, the catechol ring with an amine group attached. Noradrenaline is similar in structure to other signalling molecules used by the body, such as adrenaline and dopamine. Noradrenaline and adrenaline are both used throughout the body, but notably as part of the sympathetic nervous system and as such are often considered together.

As well as occurring naturally in the body, noradrenaline and adrenaline can also be administered to patients as medicines. Whilst they are commonly known as noradrenaline and adrenaline within the UK, they are known internationally (based upon the WHO International non-proprietary name) as norepinephrine and epinephrine. Practitioners should be familiar with both names and be aware that the literature relating to these agents and the name of products may refer to the international rather than the British names. A clear example of this is the adrenaline autoinjector used for the treatment of anaphylaxis, the best-known brand of which is the Epipen®.

Noradrenaline can sometimes be thought of as being the little brother of the better-known adrenaline. Both are the key agents through which the sympathetic nervous system

Rapid Medicines Management for Healthcare Professionals, First Edition. Paul Deslandes, Simon Young and Ben Pitcher.
© 2020 John Wiley & Sons Ltd. Published 2020 by John Wiley & Sons Ltd.

stimulates the organs and tissues of the body. The sympathetic nervous system has an impact on many organs and systems throughout the body, stimulating processes associated with increased physical activity (often referred to as 'fight or flight') and inhibiting activities associated with lower physical activity. Whilst adrenaline is released from the adrenal gland into the blood supply (and thereby affects every part of the body) noradrenaline is predominantly released from sympathetic nerve fibres directly onto tissues and organs. This allows noradrenaline to achieve selective, on-demand activation of specific systems and processes rather than the system-wide, all or nothing impact seen with adrenaline.

Noradrenaline can bind to adrenergic receptors on a variety of tissues around the body, although the action it has on different tissues can be radically different. For example, noradrenaline can cause smooth muscle contraction on the neck of the bladder, but smooth muscle relaxation in walls of the arteries supplying the muscles. These differences in action are mediated via different adrenergic receptor subtypes. These were initially grouped into two major types, alpha (α) and beta (β), but are now further divided into a number of subtypes including α_1, α_2, β_1, and β_2.

Therapeutic uses

Noradrenaline can be administered intravenously for the purposes of raising the blood pressure of a critically ill patient (this is discussed in greater depth in Chapter 41). Other drugs are used to mimic its actions (termed 'sympathomimetics') or to block its actions (e.g. beta-blockers).

Acetylcholine

Acetylcholine is used as a neurotransmitter throughout the body. It is the principal neurotransmitter of the parasympathetic nervous system, promoting activities associated with lower physical activity and reduced state of mental arousal (often described as "rest and digest"). The parasympathetic nervous system typically works in opposition to the sympathetic nervous system, creating the opposite response in a given system. Acetylcholine is also used in other distinct systems, most notably at the neuromuscular junction. When a signal is sent from a patient's brain to a muscle in order to stimulate a contraction of the muscle, it is acetylcholine that is released from the motor-neuron and binds to the receptors on the muscle cell membrane to achieve a response.

These fundamentally different functions of acetylcholine are mediated via distinctly different receptor types. Unlike adrenergic receptors, which are named after letters from the Greek alphabet, cholinergic receptor types are named after the substances which were used to characterise them. Those were muscarine and nicotine, resulting in muscarinic and nicotinic receptors, respectively. As with adrenergic receptors, both of these types are further subdivided. The distinction between muscarinic and nicotinic receptors is important and useful, as it makes it possible to block the parasympathetic actions of acetylcholine without blocking the receptors at the neuromuscular junction (which would paralyse the patient).

Therapeutic uses

Muscarinic receptors are a commonly used target for drugs, many of which are antagonists (or anti-muscarinics), which prevent acetylcholine from binding to the receptor and blocking its resulting actions. Some of the more common uses of anti-muscarinic agents include the reduction of parasympathetic nervous system mediated oral secretions and bronchoconstriction (facilitating bronchodilation). The side effects associated with antimuscarinic drugs, such as gastrointestinal disturbance and tachycardia, are a result of the disruption of the normal parasympathetic control of those body systems.

Nicotinic receptors are found throughout the body, including within the brain. It is these central nicotinic receptors that are stimulated by nicotine from tobacco, ultimately resulting in pleasurable effects. However, the peripheral nicotinic cholinergic receptors can also be therapeutic targets. Antagonists such atracurium are used to block the neuromuscular junction and paralyse a patient to prevent involuntary movements during surgery.

The effects of acetylcholine are rapidly terminated by the action of an enzyme known as acetylcholinesterase. Inhibiting this enzyme prolongs the effects of acetylcholine at its site of action, and can result in therapeutic and other effects. An example of a drug that inhibits the enzyme is donepezil (used in the treatment of dementia), whilst many nerve toxins, such as sarin, VX, and novichok, inhibit its action with fatal consequences.

4   Neurotransmitters II

In addition to the effects mediated by the autonomic nervous system (ANS), a number of physiological responses are controlled through the actions of other neurotransmitters acting at specific receptors. Like the ANS, these represent useful targets for drug action for the management of the symptoms of a number of neurological, psychological, and other illnesses. Some of the neurotransmitters most commonly targeted by available drugs include dopamine, 5-hydroxytryptamine (serotonin), endogenous opioids, and gamma-aminobutyric acid (GABA).

Dopamine

Dopamine is one of the principal neurotransmitters in the central nervous system. Dopaminergic neurons are arranged in discrete pathways in the brain and mediate effects including movement, motivation and reward, and the control of prolactin release. As a result, changes in the functioning of dopaminergic neurons can result in a number of disease states. A loss of neurons in the nigro-striatal pathway with corresponding reduced activity is associated with Parkinson's disease, whilst reduced activity in the tuberoinfundibular pathway is associated with hyperprolactinaemia. Addictive drugs and behaviours are associated with increases in activity in the mesolimbic pathway, whilst antipsychotic medicines used in the treatment of schizophrenia block dopamine D_2 receptors. Stimulation of dopamine receptors in the chemoreceptor trigger zone of the brain results in nausea and vomiting. Peripheral effects of dopamine include increased cardiac output and renal vasodilatation.

Dopamine exerts its effects through five subtypes of G-protein coupled receptor, named the dopamine D_{1-5} receptors. These receptors are grouped into two types, according to the G-proteins to which they couple. The dopamine D_1-like (including D_1 and D_5) receptors are stimulatory, coupling to G_s and increasing levels of cyclic adenosine monophosphate (cAMP). The D_2-like (including the dopamine D_2, D_3, and D_4) receptors are inhibitory, coupling to $G_{i/o}$ and reducing levels of cAMP. Currently drugs targeting D_1, D_2, and D_3 receptors as well as those promoting the formation of dopamine from its precursor levodopa (L-DOPA) are used clinically.

Dopamine is synthesised in neurons through the action of enzymes, which convert a precursor molecule (or building block) into dopamine itself. L-DOPA is a precursor of dopamine and is converted to dopamine in the brain. Once dopamine has been released from a neuron and had an effect, it is metabolised by different enzymes. By providing more of the precursor in the form of medication, or by inhibiting the metabolism of dopamine, we can increase the activity of dopamine in the brain. Increased dopamine activity can, in part, compensate for the loss of dopamine neurons seen in Parkinson's disease. Therefore medicines delivering L-DOPA, such as co-beneldopa and co-careldopa, are used in the treatment of this disorder. Reducing the metabolism of dopamine by inhibiting enzymes such as monoamine oxidase-B and catechol-O-methyl transferase with drugs such as selegiline and entacapone is an alternative approach.

Rapid Medicines Management for Healthcare Professionals, First Edition. Paul Deslandes, Simon Young and Ben Pitcher.
© 2020 John Wiley & Sons Ltd. Published 2020 by John Wiley & Sons Ltd.

Drugs stimulating dopamine D_2 receptors (e.g. bromocriptine, cabergoline, and pramipexole) also attenuate the symptoms of Parkinson's disease. However, all of these medicines may be associated with adverse effects such as nausea and vomiting, and hallucinations. Stimulation of dopamine receptors by drugs such as methylphenidate is used in the treatment of attention deficit hyperactivity disorder (ADHD). Increased dopamine activity also forms the basis of the rewarding and stimulant effects of drugs of abuse such as amfetamine and cocaine.

Drugs inhibiting dopamine receptors include the typical and atypical antipsychotics used in the treatment of schizophrenia and other psychotic illnesses. As well as helping with symptoms of psychosis, inhibiting the action of dopamine can lead to some of the adverse effects associated with these drugs, such as raised prolactin levels and Parkinsonian-type movement disorders.

5-hydroxytryptamine

5-hydroxytryptamine (5-HT) is also known as serotonin. It is important to be aware of the different terms used to describe this molecule, as each may be used in different circumstances. For example, receptors for 5-HT are named 5-HT_{1-7}, whereas the reuptake transporter protein for 5-HT is known as the serotonin reuptake transporter (SERT).

The signalling molecule 5-HT is found in the brain and also in peripheral tissues, particularly the gastrointestinal tract and blood. In the brain it helps to regulate homeostatic processes such as temperature, appetite, mood, and sleep. In the gastrointestinal tract 5-HT has both neurotransmitter and endocrine roles, and its effects include regulation of peristalsis and secretion. In the blood, 5-HT can affect blood vessels, causing either vasodilatation or vasoconstriction, depending upon the vessel and receptor present. 5-HT also has an important role in facilitating platelet aggregation.

The effects of 5-HT are mediated through a variety of different receptors, the majority of which are coupled to G-proteins, although the 5-HT_3 receptor is a ligand-gated ion channel. There are seven subgroups of 5-HT receptor (5-HT_{1-7}). A number of established medicines target the 5-HT_1, 5-HT_2, 5-HT_3, and 5-HT_4 subgroups, whilst effects at 5-HT_6 and 5-HT_7 may contribute to the action of certain medicines used in the treatment of mental illness, although their effects are less well understood.

A number of drugs target the different 5-HT receptors or the reuptake of 5-HT via the serotonin transporter to produce their therapeutic effects. Drugs acting at the 5-HT_{1A} receptor include the partial agonist buspirone (used for anxiety), whilst the 'triptans' (e.g. sumatriptan) used in migraine are agonists of $5\text{-HT}_{1B/1D}$ receptors. Many drugs used in the treatment of psychiatric disorders block the 5-HT_{2A} receptor (e.g. the antidepressants mirtazapine and mianserin and the antipsychotics risperidone and olanzapine) or the 5-HT_{2C} receptor. Blocking the 5-HT_{2A} receptor may underlie the reduction in movement disorders seen with certain atypical antipsychotic medicines, whilst blockade of the 5-HT_{2C} receptor may play a role in the increased appetite seen with antipsychotics such as olanzapine and clozapine. Antagonists of the 5-HT_3 receptor (e.g. ondansetron) are used in the treatment of nausea and vomiting, whilst 5-HT_4 receptor agonists are also used for their effects on the gastrointestinal tract. Prucalopride is a 5-HT_4 receptor agonist used in the management of constipation, whilst metoclopramide combines dopamine blocking and 5-HT_4 agonist properties and is used as an anti-emetic.

The SERT facilitates the uptake of 5-HT into the presynaptic neuron, thus helping to terminate its effect. Inhibition of the SERT is therefore a target for a number of drugs that aim to increase the effects of 5-HT in the synaptic cleft. Many antidepressants are serotonin reuptake inhibitors, including the selective serotonin reuptake inhibitors (e.g. fluoxetine and sertraline), the serotonin and noradrenaline reuptake inhibitors (e.g. duloxetine and venlafaxine), and the tricyclic antidepressants (e.g. clomipramine). Other drugs can also inhibit the reuptake of 5-HT as part of their action such as the opioid analgesic tramadol. The use of combinations of different antidepressants or other drugs inhibiting 5-HT reuptake can, in certain circumstances, lead to the serious adverse effect of serotonin syndrome.

Gamma-aminobutyric acid

The amino acid GABA is the principal inhibitory neurotransmitter in the brain. It acts through two different types of receptor, termed $GABA_A$ and $GABA_B$. $GABA_A$ receptors are chloride ion channels, and stimulation by GABA causes the channel to open, resulting in hyperpolarisation of the neuron and a reduction in activity. Through synaptic connections, GABA-containing neurons can reduce the activity of other neurons in the brain. Medicines designed to enhance the effect of GABA (and reduce neuronal activity) are useful in the treatment of conditions such as epilepsy, which are characterised by increased neuronal firing. Increasing the effect of GABA at $GABA_A$ receptors also results in an anxiolytic effect and sedation, and forms the basis of the mechanism of action of the benzodiazepines (such as diazepam and lorazepam) and Z-drugs (e.g. zopiclone). In addition to their anticonvulsant and anxiolytic effects, benzodiazepines can cause sedation and memory impairment. There are several different types of $GABA_A$ receptor, and it was hoped that targeting specific subtypes might result in drugs with fewer adverse effects. However, this is yet to be fully realised in practice.

The $GABA_B$ receptor is a G-protein coupled receptor that also has an inhibitory effect on neuronal activity. Baclofen is one of the few medicines that act at the $GABA_B$ receptor, and is used in the treatment of muscle spasticity. There has also been interest in its use in alcohol dependence.

Endogenous opioids

The endogenous opioids (or opioid peptides) are large neurotransmitter molecules found in both central and peripheral neurons. There are a number of opioid peptides present in the body, termed endorphins. These endorphins act through (and stimulate) different types of G-protein coupled opioid receptor, resulting in inhibitory effects. The most relevant receptors to drug action were originally named after the Greek letters mu (μ), delta (δ), and kappa (κ), although in a newer classification system they are known as MOPr (mu opioid receptor), DOPr (delta opioid receptor), and KOPr (kappa opioid receptor). By stimulating opioid receptors, the opioid peptides mediate a number of physiological effects in the body, one of the most important being analgesia.

Extracts from the opium poppy are able to stimulate opioid receptors in the same way as endogenous opioids and have been used for centuries for both medicinal and recreational purposes. One of the compounds found in poppy extract is morphine, which is still clinically important today. Other opioid medicines, such as pethidine, fentanyl, loperamide, and methadone, are chemically synthesised. Stimulation of opioid receptors by these medicines not only results in analgesia, but also sedation, relaxation, constipation, pupil constriction, and respiratory depression. Whilst some of these effects may be useful therapeutically (the medicine loperamide slows gastrointestinal motility and is sometimes used to treat diarrhoea), respiratory depression in particular presents a significant risk to patient safety, particularly in overdose. Another effect of stimulating opioid receptors is to induce euphoria. This forms the basis of the addictive properties of opioids, which is a significant societal problem. Drugs that block the effects of opioids (such as naloxone and naltrexone) are used in the treatment of acute overdose and in the management of opioid addiction.

5 Receptors

Many physiological effects are mediated through the action of chemical signalling molecules (such as neurotransmitters) acting in various tissues. In order for these signalling molecules to exert an effect, they must typically interact with a specific site on a target cell. A chemical signalling molecule acting at such a site is termed a ligand and the site of action is called a receptor.

Although an oversimplification, the receptor can be thought of as a switch that is able to activate or inhibit a specific action of the cell on which it is located. Following binding of the ligand to the receptor, a process (or cascade of events) is initiated, which results in a change in activity of the associated cell and a resulting physiological effect.

A number of drugs are able to act upon receptor sites found in various tissues (e.g. the cell membranes of neurons or muscle cells), and this interaction with the receptor is responsible for their therapeutic effect. The nature of the effect is determined by the type of receptor, the tissue on which the receptor is located, and the properties of the drug. Receptors therefore represent an important mechanism for mediating the effects of many drugs.

Pre- and Postsynaptic receptors and neuronal transmission

The nature of the G-protein or ligand gated ion channel to which these two types of receptor couple determines the intracellular effects mediated by activation of these receptors. However, the physiological response to receptor activation may also vary according to the location of the receptor. At the synapse, receptors may be located on either the pre- or postsynaptic neuron. Presynaptic receptors (autoreceptors) regulate neurotransmitter synthesis and release. Postsynaptic receptors (located on the postsynaptic neuron) regulate the activity of the postsynaptic neuron and the associated tissue.

Receptor types

The number of chemical signalling molecules in the body is vast, and accordingly there is a large number of receptors with which they interact. Many receptors are located in cell membranes, although some are found inside the cell cytoplasm. Receptors in the cell membrane are typically composed of a region outside the cell (the extracellular region) where the ligand is able to bind. There are also membrane-spanning and intracellular regions through which the receptor exerts an effect on the cell. When a ligand binds to the extracellular part of the receptor, it triggers a change in the intracellular region, ultimately leading to a physiological effect.

Receptors can be grouped according to the way in which they mediate a change in cellular function. They are broadly categorised into four groups: G-protein coupled receptors, ligand-gated ion channels, catalytic receptors, and nuclear receptors. Many medicines act

Rapid Medicines Management for Healthcare Professionals, First Edition. Paul Deslandes, Simon Young and Ben Pitcher.
© 2020 John Wiley & Sons Ltd. Published 2020 by John Wiley & Sons Ltd.

upon G-protein coupled receptors (e.g. salbutamol) and ligand-gated ion channels (e.g. benzodiazepines), whilst catalytic receptors are targeted by medicines such as ibrutinib, used in the treatment of certain types of cancer. Nuclear receptors include the glucocorticoid receptor, which is the target for corticosteroids such as beclometasone.

G-protein coupled receptors

These receptors are so-called because their effects are mediated through an association between the intracellular region of the receptor and a G-protein. G-proteins act as intracellular signalling molecules and once activated (by a ligand binding to the receptor) are able to bind to enzymes or ion channels in the cell to bring about a response.

There are a number of different types of G-protein which couple to different receptors. Some G-proteins can be considered excitatory (e.g. G_s) and facilitate a cascade of events within the cell, resulting in increased cyclic adenosine monophosphate (cAMP) formation. Through effects on other cellular processes, cAMP mediates increased cardiac output and smooth muscle relaxation (e.g. following activation of β_1 and β_2 adrenergic receptors, respectively). However, some G-proteins can be considered inhibitory (e.g. G_i) and reduce formation of cAMP, resulting in smooth muscle contraction (e.g. following activation of α_2 adrenoceptors). Different receptors associate with different types of G-protein, and this determines the physiological effects associated with receptor activation.

Some examples of G-protein coupled receptors are adrenergic receptors, muscarinic receptors (for the neurotransmitter acetylcholine), dopamine receptors, and many subtypes of 5-hydroxytryptamine (5-HT) receptor (for the neurotransmitter serotonin or 5-HT). Drugs acting on these receptors include salbutamol, which stimulates β_2 adrenergic receptors, and ipratropium, which inhibits muscarinic receptors, both of which cause smooth muscle relaxation and are useful in the treatment of asthma.

Ligand-gated ion channels

Some receptors mediate the opening of ion channels in the cytoplasmic membranes of nerve or muscle cells. These channels allow the movement of ions (such as sodium, potassium, calcium, or chloride) directly into or out of the cell, altering the potential difference across the membrane and thus the excitability of the cell. The resulting effect may be excitatory due to depolarisation of the cell, leading to generation of an action potential. Conversely, the effect may be inhibitory due to hyperpolarisation of the cell, reducing the likelihood of an action potential.

Channels may conduct positively charged ions (cations) such as Na^+, Ca^{2+}, K^+ or negatively charged ions (anions) such as Cl^-, and the type of ion that is conducted determines the nature of the effect. Influx of sodium and calcium via cation channels will lead to the generation of an action potential, whilst influx of chloride ions via anion channels will have an inhibitory effect. Because the receptor site directly affects the functioning of the ion channel, the effects of ligands at these receptors are mediated very quickly.

Some examples of ligand-gated ion channel receptors, their endogenous ligands and ions as well as some examples of medicines acting at the receptor are shown in Table 5.1.

Catalytic receptors

Catalytic receptors consist of an extracellular binding region for the ligand, along with an intracellular region with enzymatic activity. As with the other receptor groups, a number of different subtypes exist. However, unlike G-protein coupled receptors and ligand-gated ion channels, which are often associated with neuronal function, catalytic receptors mediate the effects of a number of proteins, such as hormones (e.g. insulin), growth factors, and cytokines (proteins associated with immunological processes) in a variety of different cell

Table 5.1 Ligand-gated ion channel receptors and examples of associated medicines.

Receptor	Endogenous ligand	Ion	Medicine
Nicotinic	Acetylcholine	Cation	Varenicline
5-HT$_3$	Serotonin	Cation	Ondansetron
NMDA	Glutamate/glycine	Cation	Memantine
AMPA	Glutamate	Cation	Perampanel
GABA$_A$	GABA	Anion	Benzodiazepines

5-HT, 5-hydroxytryptamine; NMDA, N-methyl D-aspartate; AMPA, α-amino-3-hydroxy-5-methyl-4-isoxazolepropionic acid; GABA, gamma-aminobutyric acid.

types. Activation of the receptor by the ligand may result in a variety of effects, including cellular growth, gene transcription, and synthesis of inflammatory mediators, depending upon the type of receptor.

Catalytic cytokine receptors include those for interleukins (targeted by daclizumab used in multiple sclerosis) and tumour necrosis factor (targeted by adalimumab, a monoclonal antibody used in the treatment of inflammatory conditions such as rheumatoid arthritis). Other catalytic receptors include tyrosine kinase receptors, including those for epidermal growth factor (the site of action of medicines such as gefitinib used in the treatment of non-small cell lung cancer), insulin, and platelet-derived growth factor (the site of action of sunitinib, which is used to treat certain cancers).

Nuclear receptors

Nuclear receptors are located intracellularly and regulate gene transcription. Examples of relevant types include the NR1 type located in the nucleus and which include retinoic acid (vitamin A) receptors, thyroid hormone receptors, and peroxisome proliferator-activated receptors, which bind to fatty acids and the thiazolidinedione group of antidiabetic medicines (e.g. pioglitazone). The NR3 steroid hormone receptors are located in the cytoplasm, and include androgen, oestrogen, and glucocorticoid receptors.

6   Agonists and Antagonists

The body uses chemical messengers in the form of hormones and neurotransmitters as a means of communicating and controlling systems and processes. This use of chemical messengers to control these processes provides an opportunity for us to influence physiology by either emulating or blocking the action of the chemical messenger.

- If there is a process in the body that we find useful, or wish to enhance, we can do this by flooding the system with drugs that are similar enough to the body's own chemical messenger to trigger that same response.
- If there is a process in the body which we consider unhelpful or harmful we can block the action of the chemical messenger responsible and thereby prevent it.

Receptors
Receptors are binding sites for specific molecules. Hormones and neurotransmitters will not cause an effect in every cell, they only cause a response where there is a receptor present for them to bind to. Receptors are typically complex membrane-spanning proteins containing binding sites that the hormone or neurotransmitter might bind to. There is a variety of receptor types found throughout the body, which achieve a huge variety of actions. A given cell may have many different types of receptor to facilitate different responses to different chemicals. The concept and nature of receptors is discussed in more detail in Chapter 5.

Ligands
Any chemical that can successfully bind to a receptor is called a ligand. The term ligand may refer to the body's own (endogenous) hormone or neurotransmitter, or a drug that binds to a receptor in the body.

Agonists
Typically, an endogenous ligand (such as a neurotransmitter or hormone) will bind to a receptor and stimulate a response in the associated mechanism. We describe these ligands as agonists. If a receptor is a lock and the binding site the key hole, then the agonist is the key that fits into the lock and unlocks it.

Agonists are used where there is an existing process in the body that we wish to enhance. An example of this are the opioid analgesics (e.g. morphine), which are agonists at opioid receptors. Stimulating opioid receptors with the opioid agonist results in pain relief.

It is important to remember that whilst an agonist will cause a response in the associated cellular mechanism (such as opening an ion channel or activating an enzyme) this may not necessarily mean that it creates an obvious stimulatory response in the associated system. For example, beta-2 agonists (such as salbutamol) act on receptors in the walls of the

Rapid Medicines Management for Healthcare Professionals, First Edition. Paul Deslandes, Simon Young and Ben Pitcher.
© 2020 John Wiley & Sons Ltd. Published 2020 by John Wiley & Sons Ltd.

bronchioles, for which the endogenous agonist would be adrenaline. When salbutamol binds to the beta-2 adrenergic receptor it results in activation of an enzyme (adenylate cyclase). This enzyme produces another chemical (cyclic adenosine monophosphate) that inhibits the contraction of the muscle fibres, facilitating relaxation of the muscle and bronchodilation. The agonist causes a response, but the response is the relaxation rather than contraction of the muscle.

The action of an agonist is dependent upon the cellular machinery its receptor is attached to rather than being determined by the agonist itself. As discussed above, adrenaline can stimulate the relaxation of the smooth muscle found in the bronchiolar walls. This might lead to the incorrect conclusion that adrenaline will always cause smooth muscle relaxation, but this is not the case. Adrenaline will bind to receptors on the peripheral vasculature and cause the smooth muscles to contract, causing vasoconstriction. The adrenaline does not inherently cause smooth muscle constriction or relaxation, this is determined by the nature of the receptor and its associated mechanism.

Antagonists

If an agonist is the key which unlocks the lock, then an antagonist is a key which will fit in the key hole but will not turn. An antagonist is a ligand that is capable of binding to a receptor but causes no response. Importantly, however, whilst the antagonist is bound to the receptor an agonist cannot bind and therefore the action of the agonist is blocked.

A number of different drugs act as receptor antagonists. Examples include the beta-blockers (such as atenolol and labetalol), which are a widely used treatment for hypertension. Hypertension is a disease state where blood pressure can be raised due to increased cardiac output following stimulation by the sympathetic nervous system. Adrenaline and noradrenaline are released from the adrenal medulla and the sympathetic nerve fibres, and bind to receptors on the cardiac myocytes (called beta-adrenergic receptors). These receptors, when activated, stimulate the heart to beat faster, increasing cardiac output and in turn blood pressure. Beta-blockers bind to the beta-adrenergic receptors, preventing adrenaline and noradrenaline from binding. With the adrenaline and noradrenaline unable to bind they are unable to stimulate the heart and without this stimulation the heart slows, the cardiac output drops, and the blood pressure is reduced.

Other examples

Histamine is released in response to the presence of irritants and allergens, and mediates the inflammatory response, resulting in itching and redness. Antihistamines (such as chlorphenamine) block histamine receptors, preventing the binding of histamine, and the inflammatory response (and the itching) is reduced.

Antimuscarinics (such as ipratropium) inhibit the action of the parasympathetic nervous system by blocking muscarinic acetylcholine receptors. In the lungs, acetylcholine stimulates bronchoconstriction (which makes it harder to get air into and out of the lungs). Blocking the muscarinic receptors prevents acetylcholine from causing bronchoconstriction, making breathing easier for patients with asthma or chronic obstructive pulmonary disease.

Partial agonists

Some ligands will bind to a receptor and cause a response, but a smaller response than the endogenous agonist. These are called partial agonists. They can be useful as they reduce the action of the endogenous agonist, resulting in a lesser physiological response, without completely inhibiting its effect. An example of this is oxprenolol. When it binds to the beta-adrenergic receptors, it prevents noradrenaline and adrenaline from binding and therefore reduces blood pressure. However, because it causes some response (rather than no response) it has a milder effect and reduced risk of adverse effects compared with other beta-blockers.

Super agonists

The size of the response elicited by an agonist is always compared to the size of response produced by the endogenous agonist. Whilst an agonist that produces a response smaller than the endogenous agonist is called a partial agonist, an agonist that produces a response larger than the endogenous agonist is called a super agonist. These can be used to stimulate a greater response within a given biological system than is typically seen. They may also allow a far smaller dose of drug to be used, which may facilitate the use of alternative routes of administration.

Receptor selectivity

The body uses the same chemicals (such as noradrenaline, acetylcholine, and histamine) for different purposes in different tissues throughout the body. For example, adrenaline will bind to beta-1 receptors in the heart, increasing heart rate, beta-2 receptors in the lungs, causing bronchodilation, and alpha-1 receptors, which cause constriction of the neck of prostate. These differing effects result from the presence of different receptors in the different tissues. Whilst these different receptor types all respond to the same endogenous agonist, it is possible to produce exogenous chemicals (drugs) that only work (or mostly work) on one type of receptor. Such drugs are termed selective ligands, and they allow us to target particular tissues and organs with minimal effects on others.

7 Enzymes as Drug Targets

Enzymes can be defined as protein biological catalysts. Enzymes are found in living systems, where they function to speed up biochemical reactions to support the biological system. The human body requires enzymes in order to maintain a whole range of biological processes; enzymatic actions are crucial for cellular processes such as the manufacture of proteins, DNA replication, and apoptosis. Many enzymes control the generation of energy, the breakdown of neurotransmitters, and the control of critical homeostatic mechanisms such as blood pressure, coagulation, and body temperature. Having well-defined structures, enzymes are an ideal drug target.

Enzymes as targets for drug action

If there is an enzymatically controlled process in the body that leads to a pathological change, an enzyme inhibitor may be used to prevent the enzyme from working and alter the course of that biochemical pathway. For example, angiotensin-converting enzyme (ACE) is part of a complex biological process that maintains and raises blood pressure. If a patient is hypertensive, ACE inhibitor drugs can be given (which prevent the enzyme from exerting its catalytic action) and the result is a fall in blood pressure. Inhibiting the enzyme cyclooxygenase (with non-steroidal anti-inflammatory drugs such as ibuprofen) results in a reduction in inflammation that is useful in the management of pain and conditions such as rheumatoid arthritis.

Classification and nomenclature of enzymes

There are hundreds of thousands of different enzymes. Their names often illustrate what function the enzyme performs. Enzyme names usually end in -ase, for example ATP synthase 'constructs' a chemical called ATP, DNA polymerase 'reads' a DNA strand and uses it as a template to make a new strand, and amylase facilities the breakdown of starch. Enzymes can also be labelled as groups or families, e.g. proteases break down other enzymes and proteins into amino acids.

When considering the actions of enzymes some serve to break large chemicals into smaller chemicals, others take smaller chemicals and build them up into bigger chemicals, and others undertake many other vital biochemical tasks. The classification below lists the main types.

Enzymes are classified by the International Union of Biochemistry into six classes:

1. *Oxido-reductases*: catalyse the transfer of electrons.
2. *Transferases*: shift chemical functional groups from one molecule to another.
3. *Hydrolases*: add and an –OH (hydroxyl) group to a molecule.
4. *Lyases*: split chemical bonds.

Rapid Medicines Management for Healthcare Professionals, First Edition. Paul Deslandes, Simon Young and Ben Pitcher.
© 2020 John Wiley & Sons Ltd. Published 2020 by John Wiley & Sons Ltd.

5. *Isomerases*: 'flip' chemicals between isomeric forms. Isomers are two or more compounds with the same formula but a different arrangement of atoms in the molecule and different properties.
6. *Ligases*: typically join two large molecules.

How do they work?

Enzymes are long strings of amino acids that can form into complex three-dimensional structures. The specific orientation and type of amino acids in the structure create an active site for a specific type of molecule, termed the substrate, to bind. The enzyme will then transform the substrate into the product.

The general equation for an enzymatic reaction is:

$$substrate + enzyme \rightarrow substrate - enzyme \rightarrow product - enzyme \rightarrow product + enzyme.$$

The substrate binds with the enzyme to form a substrate–enzyme complex, then as the reaction progresses the product of the reaction forms a complex with the enzyme and finally the enzyme and the product(s) separate. Note that the enzyme is unchanged by the reaction.

Example

Sucrase splits sucrose into its constituent sugars (glucose and fructose). The sucrase 'bends' the sucrose and strains the bond between the glucose and fructose. Water molecules assist and break (cleave) the bond in a fraction of a second.

Enzymes have these key features:

- They are catalytic.
- They can increase reaction rates a billion-fold or more.
- They are effective in very small quantities. One enzyme molecule may convert thousands of substrates in few seconds.
- They are highly specific. One enzyme will typically only carry out one specific role or task (this makes them ideal drug targets).

Enzyme inhibition

Enzymes can be inhibited in a reversible or irreversible manner.

Reversible inhibitors

Reversible inhibitors bind to enzymes in relatively weak fashion and can be easily removed by altering the environment of the reaction. This means that when a reversible inhibitor is used as a drug there is rapid cycling of the inhibitor blocking the enzyme and the enzyme being available to catalyse its reaction. Reversible inhibitors can be divided into three subtypes.

Competitive inhibitors

These inhibitors compete with the substrate for the enzymatic binding site. Increasing the amount of substrate helps overcome this inhibition. For example, warfarin is a competitive inhibitor of the enzyme vitamin K epoxide reductase, for which vitamin K is the normal substrate. Increasing the amount of available vitamin K will overcome the inhibition and reverse the action of warfarin.

Uncompetitive inhibitors
These bind to the enzyme but instead of binding to the active site, the inhibitor binds at a location that interferes with the ability of the substrate to bind to the active site (but does not prevent it). Increasing the concertation of the substrate reduces the degree of inhibition but does not eliminate it. The mood stabiliser lithium is an uncompetitive inhibitor of inositol monophosphatase.

Non-competitive inhibitors
These inhibitors bind to other sites on the enzyme, not the active site. These sites are termed allosteric sites. The disruption of the active site by the allosteric binding means that this inhibition cannot be overcome or reduced by increasing the concentration of the substrate. For example, the drug acetazolamide inhibits the carbonic anhydrase enzyme in a non-competitive manner.

Irreversible (suicide) inhibitors
This group bind very strongly to an enzyme and permanently change the active site of that enzyme. This process cannot be chemically reversed.

Suicide inhibitors are also known as mechanism-based inhibitors. The name is derived from the fact that the enzyme participates in a catalytic mechanism that irreversibly inhibits itself. These inhibitors are substrates that have been modified. Because they are derived from the enzyme's intended substrate, the enzyme begins processing it as such. However, as catalysis progresses, the modifications of the substrate result in a reactive intermediate that forms covalent bonds with the enzyme that irreversibly inactivates it.

Some clinical examples of suicide inhibitors include aspirin (which inhibits cyclooxygenase 1 and 2 enzymes) and clavulanic acid (which inhibits β-lactamase, permanently inactivating it and 'protecting' the co-administered amoxicillin antibacterial agent).

8 Transport Proteins and Channels

Drugs can exert their action through a variety of different mechanisms. These include via receptors or through the interference with the normal function of enzymes, as discussed in Chapters 5 and 7, respectively. Another avenue for drug action is to directly act upon the transport proteins that would normally facilitate the movement of substances (such as ions) from one side of the cell membrane to the other. This mechanism forms the focus of this chapter.

The cell membrane

The cell membrane provides a barrier to the movement of substances into and out of the cell, allowing it to maintain homeostasis. Similar membranes may also be found within the cell, surrounding internal stores of various substances, as well as mitochondria and the cell nucleus.

The membrane is composed of a phospholipid bilayer, which creates a hydrophobic layer that prevents water and water-soluble substances (e.g. glucose, Na^+, K^+, and Cl^-) from entering or leaving the cell. The movement of these substances must therefore be facilitated via a variety of transmembrane proteins such as channels and transporters.

Transmembrane proteins

Proteins are polypeptides, long strings of amino acids that can form complex three-dimensional shapes. Different amino acids within the polypeptide chain can have varying degrees of water or lipid solubility. This can create proteins where some sections of the structure are lipid soluble and other regions are water soluble. The lipid-soluble regions of a protein can become embedded in the lipid membrane, whilst the water-soluble regions will remain in either the cytosol or extracellular fluid. If a protein has regions which are in the extracellular fluid, within the cell membrane, and in the cytosol then it can be described as a membrane-spanning protein.

These membrane-spanning proteins can be grouped together to form complex structures such as channels, which can provide an opening in the cell membrane to allow substances to move from one side to the other. The shape of these structures can shift from one conformational arrangement to another, essentially opening or closing the channel or even actively transporting a substance from one side to the other. These changes in conformation can be triggered by the binding of substances to the transmembrane protein or a change in the environment (such as a change in the membrane voltage that forms part of the depolarisation of a cell).

Rapid Medicines Management for Healthcare Professionals, First Edition. Paul Deslandes, Simon Young and Ben Pitcher.
© 2020 John Wiley & Sons Ltd. Published 2020 by John Wiley & Sons Ltd.

Channels

There are many examples of drugs that act on ion channels, which when open allow ions to flow through a pore in the centre of the channel and across the cell membrane along the concentration gradient. Lidocaine (and other local anaesthetics) block the voltage-gated sodium channels on neurons. These typically open in response to a change in membrane voltage, allowing an influx of Na^+ ions, which continue the propagation of the action potential along the axon. By physically obstructing the ion channel, drugs such as lidocaine prevent the continuation of the action potential and thereby prevent the transmission of sensation, blocking pain.

Similarly, calcium channel blockers (e.g. amlodipine, diltiazem) disrupt the movement of calcium ions across the cellular membrane through L-type voltage-gated ion channels. Blocking this calcium influx prevents the release of calcium from the cell's internal stores and reduces activity within the cell. In vascular smooth muscle this prevents muscle contraction and causes vasodilation. In cardiac myocytes it reduces contraction and electrical conduction.

Transporters

Transport proteins can facilitate the movement of substances across cell membranes in a more regulated fashion. This can be along the concentration gradient or be a form of active transport, utilising energy to move substances against the concentration gradient. There are many drugs that act upon these transporters and thereby prevent this movement of specific substances.

The parietal cells in the lining of the stomach use the transporter $H^+/K^+/ATPase$ to move or 'pump' acidifying hydrogen ions (protons) into the stomach, creating stomach acid. Proton pump inhibitors (PPIs) such as omeprazole or lansoprazole inhibit the proton pump ($H^+/K^+/ATPase$) and thereby prevent the secretion of acid into the stomach and therefore raise stomach pH.

Some transport proteins are involved in the reuptake of neurotransmitters from the synaptic cleft back into the neuron. This is part of the process through which a synapse is reset after a successful synaptic transmission. Selective serotonin re-uptake inhibitors such as fluoxetine prevent this reuptake and thereby facilitate higher levels of serotonin in the synaptic cleft thereby increasing its effect.

Receptor-mediated ion channels

This chapter has described ion channels and transport proteins as a separate pharmacological target to receptors. However, there are circumstances where the difference between these pharmacological targets becomes less distinct. Receptor-mediated (sometimes also called ligand-gated) ion channels open in response to the binding of an agonist to allow the movement of ions into or out of the cell. These are discussed in greater depth in Chapter 5.

Indirect influence on transport proteins

Some drugs can have an indirect action on transport proteins even if their own principal pharmacological action is different. For example, ranitidine is a histamine H_2 receptor antagonist. It prevents histamine from activating a cellular process, resulting in the $H^+/K^+/$ATPase transporter not being utilised. The end result is that the transport protein's action is inhibited. However, the action of the drug is still a receptor antagonist and is distinct from the action of the PPIs, which act directly on the $H^+/K^+/ATPase$ itself.

9 Hormones

Hormones are members of a group of signalling molecules/chemical messengers that are excreted by endocrine glands. Hormones are typically transported to their site of action by the circulatory system. Their target site of action is often distant from their site of production and excretion (compare with neurotransmitters). Hormones typically control physiological process but can also influence behaviour (Table 9.1).

When considering pharmacological interventions, the drug entities utilised in clinical practice often interact with neurotransmitters (and their function), ion channels or enzymes. Intervening to change these systems often restores homeostasis or corrects pathophysiologic dysfunction. However, some medications used in practice also include substances that alter the effects of, mimic the effects of or replace hormones (Table 9.2).

Hormone classes

Hormones in humans fall into three broad biochemical categories:

1. amino acid/peptide/protein derived, e.g. thyroxine, insulin
2. eicosanoids, e.g. prostaglandins
3. steroids, e.g. oestrogen, testosterone, and aldosterone.

Many other examples can be found of medication that interacts with hormone pathways. Table 9.2 gives a summary of the commonly encountered hormonal interventions.

Rapid Medicines Management for Healthcare Professionals, First Edition. Paul Deslandes, Simon Young and Ben Pitcher.
© 2020 John Wiley & Sons Ltd. Published 2020 by John Wiley & Sons Ltd.

Table 9.1 Hormone-producing glands.

Gland that produces the hormone	Example(s) of a hormone produced by the gland	Function of the hormone
Adrenal	Aldosterone	Mineralocorticoids – regulation of mineral balance
	Adrenaline (epinephrine)	A component of the sympathetic nervous system (stress hormone)
	Androgens	Precursors to male sex hormones
	Cortisol/hydrocortisone	Glucocorticoids – regulation of glucose metabolism (stress hormone)
Hypothalamus	'Releasing hormones' that control the release of hormones in other parts of the body, e.g. the anterior pituitary	The hypothalamus is responsible for controlling body temperature, hunger, mood, and the release of hormones from other glands, and also controls thirst, sleep, and sex drive
Ovaries	Oestrogen and progesterone	Female sex hormones
Pancreas	Insulin and glucagon (and other hormones, e.g. somatostatin)	Glucose homeostasis
Parathyroid	Parathyroid hormone	This gland controls calcium homeostasis in the body and bone remodelling
Pineal	Melatonin	Influences circadian rhythm and sleep/wake cycles
Pituitary	Adrenocorticotropic hormone, follicle-stimulating hormone growth hormone, prolactin, and thyroid-stimulating hormone	Theses hormones control and regulate the function of other endocrine glands
Testes	Androgens, e.g. testosterone	Male sex hormones
Thyroid	Triiodothyronine T_3 and thyroxine T_4	Control rate of metabolic processes, cardiovascular parameters, and development/growth rate
	Calcitonin	Calcium metabolism (opposing the effects of parathyroid hormone)
Thymus	Thymosin	T-cell development

Table 9.2 Examples of hormones used in medicinal interventions.

Example(s) of a hormone	Examples of medicines that mimic or block the effect of the hormone	Noted indication for the use of the medication	Notes
Aldosterone	Medications such as spironolactone and eplerenone block (antagonise) the effects of aldosterone	Lower blood pressure in resistant hypertension, treat the symptoms of heart failure and used for ascites	Causes potassium retention, leading to hyperkalaemia
Adrenaline (epinephrine)	Beta-2 receptor agonists mimic the action of adrenaline in the lungs, causing bronchodilation	Asthma, bronchoconstriction	
	Beta-blockers such as atenolol block the effects of adrenaline	Angina, hypertension, heart failure, and ar-rhythmias	
Androgens	Testosterone (a copy of the body's natural hormone)	Hypogonadism due to testosterone deficiency in men	
Cortisol/hydrocortisone (often referred to as 'steroids')	Hydrocortisone (a copy of the body's natural hormone)	Wide range of uses from skin conditions such as eczema to hormone deficiency such as Addison's disease Control autoimmune and inflammatory diseases	Hydrocortisone is available in a range of formulations for a variety of indications, e.g. cream, ointment, tablets, and injectable forms
Oestrogen and progesterone	Combined oral contraceptives contain analogues of oestrogen and progesterone, e.g. Marvelon® (ethinylestradiol 30 micrograms and desogestrel 150 micrograms)	Hormonal contraception	Oestrogen and progesterone analogues are used for contraception and hormone replacement therapy
Glucagon	Human glucagon produced by recombinant DNA technology	Insulin-induced hypoglycaemia	

(Continued)

Table 9.2 (Continued)

Example(s) of a hormone	Examples of medicines that mimic or block the effect of the hormone	Noted indication for the use of the medication	Notes
Insulin	Synthetic insulin, e.g. Actrapid® and Insulin Glargine®	Treatment of diabetes mellitus (essential for survival for type I diabetics) and often used for therapy in type II diabetics	Injectable forms only
Parathyroid hormone	Parathyroid hormone is produced by recombinant DNA technology	Parathyroid hormone controls calcium homeostasis in the body and bone remodelling	
Melatonin	Medicines that contain melatonin mimic its endogenous effects	Used to treat insomnia	Available as Circadin® 2 mg prolonged-release tablets
	Agomelatine is a melatonin receptor agonist	Depression	Valdoxan® tablets
Triiodothyronine (T_3) and thyroxine (T_4)	Medication is available containing the hormones triiodothyronine T_3 and thyroxine T_4	Used to treat hypothyroidism	
Calcitonin	An analogue (calcitonin, SALMON) is available as a medicinal product	Hypercalcaemia of malignancy Paget's disease of bone Prevention of acute bone loss due to sudden immobility	

10 Introduction to Pharmacokinetics

Pharmacokinetics is often described as 'what the body does to the drug'. It is the study of how a drug enters the body, how it is metabolised and how it is removed from the body. An understanding of pharmacokinetics allows us to understand why a drug is given by a specific route or why some drugs are given once a day and others three times a day.

ADME

When looking at pharmacokinetics we divide it into four areas, which are characterised in the letters ADME:

- **A**bsorption
- **D**istribution
- **M**etabolism
- **E**limination

Absorption: how the drug gets into the body

Absorption describes all of the different processes through which a drug gets into the body, and all of the various factors that can influence this. This includes the effectiveness or necessity of using different routes of administration as well as specific circumstances that can affect absorption.

For example, when we use medicines orally there are often instructions pertaining to when the drug should be taken in relation to food. Sometimes this should be a specific number of hours before food, sometimes after, and sometimes with. These instructions are due to the potential for food to affect how much of the drug is absorbed.

Bioavailability

When we swallow a tablet, some of the drug is broken down by digestive enzymes or by the harsh acidic environment of the stomach. When we apply a cream, not all of the drug is absorbed. When we use an inhaler, some of the drug we breathe in gets breathed back out. Most of the time, when we administer a drug not all of it reaches the systemic blood supply. The bioavailability of a drug describes what proportion of the drug does reach the systemic circulation. If a 100 mg tablet is swallowed and only 50 mg reaches the blood supply we say it has a bioavailability of 50%. Drugs administered intravenously (directly into the blood) have a bioavailability of 100%.

Rapid Medicines Management for Healthcare Professionals, First Edition. Paul Deslandes, Simon Young and Ben Pitcher.
© 2020 John Wiley & Sons Ltd. Published 2020 by John Wiley & Sons Ltd.

Distribution: how the drug gets around the body

The human body is not a hollow vessel. When we add a drug into the system it does not instantaneously distribute itself equally throughout the body. The body is made up of a variety of different compartments and tissues (e.g. blood, muscle, fat) that the drug can seep into. Some compartments are easier for the drug to access than others, which can provide a challenge for delivering drugs to specific areas.

Lipid solubility

An important factor that affects how a drug is distributed around the body is whether the drug is lipid soluble or water soluble. Lipids are fats, and they are a major constituent of cell membranes. The more lipid soluble a drug is, the easier it will be for it to move out of the bloodstream and into cells. Substances which are lipid soluble can be referred to by a number of terms, such as lipophilic or non-polar, whereas water-soluble drugs may be referred to as lipophobic, hydrophilic or polar. The brain and central nervous system is protected by a lipid-based protective barrier (known as the blood–brain barrier) that helps to protect the brain from toxins. For a drug to reach the brain and therefore have any effect there, it must be lipid soluble.

Metabolism: how the body deals with the drug

The body will treat a drug the same way that it would treat any foreign chemical. It will try to render the drug inactive, preventing it from causing any effect and making it easier to remove from the body. When we think of drug metabolism we often think about the idea of breaking drugs down. Whilst this is true for some drugs, a large part of drug metabolism is actually adding to the drug molecule. By adding large water-soluble conjugates to the drug it becomes less lipid soluble and more water soluble. The less lipid soluble the drug becomes the harder it is for it to enter the tissues and the easier it is to be eliminated by the kidneys. However, it is important to remember that not all drugs are metabolised and some can be eliminated from the body unchanged.

Pro-drugs

Some drugs are administered in an inactive form and actually rely upon the body's metabolising processes to change them from the inactive form into the active form. These drugs are called pro-drugs. Sometimes the pro-drug is administered because it is more readily absorbed than the active form of the drug, allowing a higher bioavailability.

Elimination: how the drug gets out of the body

Whether the drug is metabolised or not, it must be removed from the body. The main route of elimination (which is sometimes called *excretion*) is via the kidneys in the urine. However, drugs can be eliminated from the body by other routes as well (such as in the faeces, sweat, and breath). The speed at which a drug is cleared from the body is reasonably predictable. This, in combination with our understanding of metabolism, allows us to predict how long a drug will remain in the body and therefore how long it will continue to have an effect.

Half-life

When discussing the elimination of drugs we often refer to half-life. This is the amount of time that it takes for the concentration of the drug in the body to reduce by half.

Imagine you administered 100 mg of a drug intravenously to a patient and after one hour the patient's body had eliminated 50 mg of the drug. You can see that in one hour the amount of the drug has halved, so its half-life is one hour. After a further hour the amount of drug would be reduced by another half, reducing the amount of drug left in the body from 50 to 25 mg. In the first hour, the amount of drug was reduced by 50 mg as this was half of the original amount. In the second hour the amount of the drug was reduced by 25 mg. This is less than in the first hour but is still half of the amount of the drug which was there. In the next hour, the quantity of drug would half again to 12.5 mg and in another hour reduce to 6.25 mg.

In general, we say that a drug will be effectively cleared from the body in five half-lives. We also say that a drug will take five half-lives to reach a steady state when it is being initiated. In the example above, the half-life was one hour so five half-lives would be five hours. However, it is important to remember that different drugs have different half-lives, which can range from seconds to weeks in length.

11 Absorption

The absorption of a drug describes its movement from outside the body through tissues and into the blood. This movement usually occurs by diffusion of the drug through the cell membranes or through the gaps between the cells which form the tissues lining the area of the body to which the drug has been administered. This is typically the endothelial cells of the buccal membrane of the mouth, the gastrointestinal (GI) tract (including the intestine and rectum), the lung, the skin, the vagina, and subcutaneous and muscle tissue. The drug may need to move across multiple cell membranes before it can reach the site of action or the blood, which will transport it around the body. It will then need to move across more membranes to leave the blood and enter the tissues where it is needed. How easily the drug can cross the cell membrane can be impacted by how lipid soluble it is. The specific chemistry of the drug is the primary dictator of this, but it can be influenced by factors such as the pH of the environment. Some drugs may be able to enter cells by travelling through ion channels or even by using active transport mechanisms.

Understanding the principles of absorption can help us to understand the effectiveness or necessity of using different routes of administration. It can also highlight specific circumstances (such as disease states or the use of other medication) that can affect absorption. For example, when we use medications orally there are often instructions pertaining to when the drug should be taken in relation to food. Sometimes this is a specific number of hours before food, sometimes after food, and sometimes with food (as this will impact on the pH of the stomach). These instructions are required because of the potential for food to affect how much of the drug is absorbed into the body.

Are all drugs absorbed in the same way?

The chemical and structural nature of a drug will affect how quickly and completely it will be absorbed via any given route. Some drugs may be absorbed easily through any route, others may be very poorly absorbed and will require routes that deliver the drug directly into the bloodstream.

The easiest way to get a drug into a patient is for them to swallow it. It is after all the purpose of the GI tract to take substances from the outside world and internalise them for use within the body. The small intestine has a large surface area, which facilitates the absorption of many drugs. However, the oral route can be slow, and it is sometimes necessary for us to get drugs into patients very quickly. In these situations we opt for alternative routes of administration such as intravenous injection. An example is the use of intravenous antibiotics for the treatment of severe infection.

Furthermore, drugs administered via the oral route may be destroyed by the harsh nature of the GI tract and the process known as first-pass metabolism. It is because of this that some drugs cannot be administered orally and must be given by parenteral (non-oral) means. For example, insulin cannot be taken orally as its protein structure is broken down by digestive enzymes. It is therefore given by either intravenous or subcutaneous injection.

Rapid Medicines Management for Healthcare Professionals, First Edition. Paul Deslandes, Simon Young and Ben Pitcher.
© 2020 John Wiley & Sons Ltd. Published 2020 by John Wiley & Sons Ltd.

What is first-pass metabolism?

When chemicals are absorbed from the GI tract into the bloodstream they are first carried through the liver. One of the functions of the liver is to detoxify our blood, metabolising and rendering safe potentially harmful substances. This is ideal for protecting us from toxins we may have inadvertently eaten, but can also dramatically reduce the amount of active drug that reaches the general circulation; this is the basis of first-pass metabolism.

What is bioavailability?

When we swallow a tablet, some of the drug is broken down by digestive enzymes or by the harsh acidic environment of the stomach. When we apply a cream, not all of the drug is absorbed. When we use an inhaler some of the drug we breathe in gets breathed back out. Most of the time when we administer a drug not all of it reaches the systemic blood supply. The bioavailability of a drug describes what proportion of the drug actually reaches the systemic circulation. If a 100 mg tablet is swallowed and only 50 mg reaches the blood supply we say it has a bioavailability of 50%. Most routes of administration have a bioavailability lower than 100%. However, drugs administered intravenously (injected directly into the blood) can achieve a bioavailability of 100%. It is important to remember, however, that reaching the bloodstream is not necessarily the same as reaching the site of action. The drug will usually still have to travel from the blood into the tissues where it will take effect.

What can affect absorption?

In the case of the oral route, many things can affect how the drug is absorbed. Medications are often formulated with a specific level of stomach acidity in mind. Instructions regarding whether to take the drug with, before or after food are often intended to help ensure the acidity within the stomach is appropriate. Any other drugs that the patient is taking to reduce acidity may therefore affect absorption.

If the anatomical structures involved in absorption are disrupted then absorption will be affected. Nausea and vomiting will reduce (or even prevent) oral absorption, whilst the motility of the GI tract, blood flow to the intestine, and the presence of other drugs (with resulting drug interactions) can also affect absorption. Absorption of drugs from other sites can also be affected, for example respiratory disease can reduce entry and absorption of inhaled medications, whilst broken or damaged skin can increase the absorption of topically applied agents.

12 Distribution

Following the process of absorption of the drug (or in the case of an intravenously administered medication, its direct injection into the circulatory system) the drug needs to be transported to its site of action in order to exert its therapeutic effect. Drugs given systemically will be distributed to their site of action via the circulatory system.

The distribution of a drug via the circulation allows drug molecules to be delivered wherever blood flows. This is advantageous as the bloodstream can rapidly deliver drugs to all parts of the body, especially those parts that receive a rich supply of blood. However, there are unfortunately several disadvantages, for example parts of the body that are not so richly perfused with blood often do not receive a rich supply of the drug (e.g. the bones). Delivering adequate drug to these sites of action can require alternative dosing strategies in order to influence the disease process. Another disadvantage is that the administered drug will be distributed to most parts of the body indiscriminately. This may include parts of the body where the drug is not needed as they are not affected by the disease process that requires treatment. However, the drug may still exert an effect on this tissue or organ, which may result in some of the adverse reactions that patients suffer when receiving drug treatment.

How do drugs move into different tissues?

The extent to which a drug can be transferred from the blood into different tissues is largely dependent upon how easily it can dissolve in water (known as hydrophilicity) and how easily it can dissolve in lipid or fat (known as lipophilicity). Drugs that are hydrophilic are less able to cross cell membranes and must pass between cells to move between different parts of the body. This makes it harder for them to enter certain organs such as the brain. Drugs that are more lipid soluble are more easily able to cross cell membranes and enter certain tissues. Lipophilicity can also allow drugs to enter liver cells, where they are exposed to metabolic enzymes that convert them into more water-soluble metabolites to facilitate elimination by the kidney. The movement of some drugs can be facilitated by transport proteins (e.g. *p*-glycoprotein), which may allow the drug to cross a membrane despite being hydrophilic or may remove a drug from a certain tissue despite it being lipophilic.

The brain

The brain is a particularly delicate organ and can easily be damaged by the presence of chemicals, including drugs. In order to protect it from the threat that drugs represent, there is a complex structure of blood vessels that prevent the movement of medication (and other substances) into the brain. This is known as the blood–brain barrier.

The blood–brain barrier, whilst providing a protective shield to prevent the ingress of unwanted drugs, may also prevent drugs that are needed from getting into the central nervous system to exert their effect. This is an important consideration when designing

Rapid Medicines Management for Healthcare Professionals, First Edition. Paul Deslandes, Simon Young and Ben Pitcher.
© 2020 John Wiley & Sons Ltd. Published 2020 by John Wiley & Sons Ltd.

drugs such as antidepressants, hypnotics, and antipsychotics, which must be able to cross the blood–brain barrier to exert their therapeutic effects. In order to cross the blood–brain barrier, drugs must be designed chemically to dissolve in lipid (they must be lipophilic).

Other useful drugs that may be prevented from entering the brain by the blood–brain barrier include certain antibiotics. Whilst the blood–brain barrier may prevent antibiotics from entering under normal physiological conditions, inflammation associated with infections such as meningitis can disrupt the integrity of the barrier. This disruption can allow the antibiotics to enter the brain and kill the invading pathogens.

The placenta

The placenta is a similar barrier to the distribution of drugs and other substances to the blood–brain barrier. It can prevent medication from being distributed from the mother to the developing foetus, where it may cause harm. However, many drugs are able to cross the placental barrier and exert an effect on the foetus, which may include a number of negative influences on health and development.

Free drug and bound drug

Drugs that are dissolved in plasma are able to pass from the bloodstream into tissues and organs to exert their effect. Pharmacokinetically, a drug that is dissolved in plasma is termed free drug, i.e. the drug is free to move from the plasma into the fluid that surrounds tissues and organs. From here, the drug can move into the tissues and organs themselves (which are typically the site of action) to exert its therapeutic effect.

In many cases, not all of the drug that is present in the bloodstream is free drug. Some drugs, because of their physicochemical properties, become attached to the dissolved proteins in the blood such as albumin and alpha-1-acid glycoprotein. Drug that is attached to plasma protein is termed bound drug. Bound drug is essentially loosely chemically attached to the protein and is unable to freely diffuse from the bloodstream into tissue that it is targeting to exert its therapeutic effect. As a result, for the drug to exert its influence at the site of action it must first uncouple from the plasma protein to become free drug.

If a drug's properties mean that it can bind to plasma proteins, then a balance is established between the amount of drug that is bound to the plasma protein and the amount that is free. Anything that upsets this balance, such as a change in the plasma protein concentration (which can be caused by conditions such as hepatic dysfunction or, burns) or the administration of two or more drugs that have the ability to bind to plasma proteins, can influence the effectiveness of the medication. In some cases (such as reduced plasma protein concentration) this may require an adjustment in drug dosing.

13 Metabolism

Introduction

In order to facilitate the removal of drugs from the body, they can be subject to significant biochemical transformations. The human body has capacity to modify the chemical structure of drugs by a process known as drug metabolism. Enzymes (protein biological catalysts) are responsible for catalysing these metabolic processes at the cellular level. The liver is the organ that carries out the majority of drug metabolism in the body, and it contains a number of different metabolic enzymes. Other organs and tissues, such as the gastrointestinal wall, kidneys, plasma, and placenta, also possess the enzymes and therefore have the capacity to undertake drug metabolism.

When a drug is administered orally it passes into the gastrointestinal tract and is absorbed into the bloodstream via the hepatic portal vein and the liver. Prior to the drug getting to the bloodstream this movement or passage through the liver and gastrointestinal wall exposes the drug to the enzyme and serves to metabolise it. This process is designed to protect the body from potentially toxic chemicals, and is known as first-pass metabolism. Some drugs do not survive this first pass and are completely transformed by the enzyme into chemicals that do not exert any pharmacological effect (these drugs are not suitable for oral administration and must be delivered to the body via an alternative route). Other drugs take this first pass totally unchanged. The majority of drugs undergo some degree of metabolism before they are allowed into general circulation. Medications administered by the oral, nasogastric, and percutaneous endoscopic gastrostomy routes will be subject to first-pass metabolism.

When the drug reaches the general circulation, it flows with the blood around the body. As the blood circulates through the liver the drug will be exposed to further metabolism by the liver. If a drug undergoes metabolism (note that not all drugs have a chemical structure that enzyme systems can detoxify) more of the drug molecules will be transformed each time they pass through the liver.

Phase I and II metabolism

Metabolism is in essence an indiscriminate biochemical transformation. There are two types of chemical reactions that occur and they are described by the terms phase I and phase II metabolism. Drugs may undergo phase I metabolism alone, phase II metabolism alone or a combination of both phases in order that the body may facilitate their elimination. As previously stated, some drugs do not undergo metabolic transformation and are eliminated from the body unchanged.

Phase I metabolic transformations are quite basic chemical reactions. They can broadly be thought of as catabolic, involving the breakdown or removal of part of the drug molecule. The metabolic enzymes perform simple chemical processes such as the addition or removal of oxygen, hydrogen, and other simple molecules such as the as the hydroxyl ion (OH^-). The cytochrome P450 isoenzyme family (commonly termed CYP or CYP450) is a key set of

Rapid Medicines Management for Healthcare Professionals, First Edition. Paul Deslandes, Simon Young and Ben Pitcher.

metabolic enzymes that are responsible for phase I transformations. When drugs have undergone phase I reactions they typically become more water soluble (more easy to eliminate) or are further prepared for phase II transformations. Each time a drug undergoes a phase I transformation it typically becomes more pharmacologically inert.

Phase II processes add larger molecules to the drug's structure (conjugation) and can therefore be broadly considered anabolic. Like phase I reactions, these phase II processes are enzyme mediated. The molecules added include glucuronic acid and sulphates, and the enzyme groups responsible include uridine 5'-diphospho-glucuronosyltransferase. The addition of these molecules to the drug structure increases the drug's water solubility significantly to facilitate elimination.

Changes (increases or decreases) in the activity of the enzyme groups responsible for phase I and phase II metabolism may contribute to variation in patient response to treatment, and also form the basis of many drug interactions (see Chapters 14 and 30). An understanding of these processes is important in predicting the dosing requirements of many medicines.

Drug activity: prodrugs

In addition to facilitating the removal of drugs from the body, the process of metabolism can affect the pharmacological activity of a drug. There are some drugs that are pharmacologically inert until they are metabolised; these are known as prodrugs. These drugs cannot exert their pharmacological action until they have undergone biochemical transformation. The International Union of Pure and Applied Chemistry (IUPAC) definition of prodrugs is that they can be '…viewed as drugs containing specialized nontoxic protective groups used in a transient manner to alter or to eliminate undesirable properties in the parent molecule' (Vert et al. 2012). The development of drugs as prodrugs may help to reduce toxicity and optimise the therapeutic effect. Prodrugs can be 'activated' intra- or extracellularly. Examples of drugs activated intracellularly include aciclovir, levodopa, and mitomycin. Examples of those activated extracellularly include fosphenytoin, lisdexamfetamine, and aspirin.

Whilst metabolism may convert inactive prodrugs into active entities, some drugs (such as the antidepressant fluoxetine) that already have pharmacological activity are themselves metabolised to chemicals that have a pharmacological effect. In this instance, the 'active drug' has an 'active metabolite'. Here, both the original drug and the active metabolite play a role in the therapeutic effect of the medication and the active metabolite may itself be further metabolised by the actions of enzymes in the liver and other tissues.

Reference

Vert, M., Doi, Y., Hellwich, K.-H. et al. (2012). Terminology for biorelated polymers and applications (IUPAC Recommendations 2012) (PDF). Pure and Applied Chemistry 84 (2): 377–410. https://doi.org/10.1351/PAC-REC-10-12-04.

14 Cytochrome P450 Enzyme Inhibitors and Inducers

The cytochrome P450 (CYP450) isoenzyme family is a group of enzymes that are responsible for facilitating many processes in the human body. In Chapter 13 on metabolism, we read about the role these enzymes play in drug metabolism (the conversion of a drug into a form that can be more easily eliminated from the body). The CYP450 group of enzymes are responsible for phase I metabolism, which affects many of the drugs that we use. There are more than 50 members of the cytochrome family, and six of these enzymes play a role in metabolising 90% of clinically used drugs. The most important members of the family are CYP3A4 and CYP2D6.

In addition to their therapeutic effects, some drugs (and other chemicals) are able to influence the activity of some of the CYP450 enzymes and interfere with their role in metabolism. These drugs can be classified as enzyme inducers (which increase the activity of CYP450 enzymes) and enzyme inhibitors (which reduce the activity of CYP450 enzymes).

Cytochrome P450 enzyme inducers

The anticonvulsant carbamazepine is a classic example of a CYP450 enzyme inducer. Carbamazepine induces the CYP3A4 type enzymes in the liver and other parts of the body (such as the gastrointestinal tract). The process of induction 'enhances' or increases the activity of the enzyme, making it more efficient at modifying the drugs that it metabolises. As a result, the amount of the affected drug in the body can be decreased, which may lead to treatment failure.

Example: carbamazepine's effect on the efficacy of combined hormonal contraceptives

Carbamazepine induces the activity of the enzyme that metabolises the combined oral contraceptive pill. The enzyme's ability to metabolise the contraceptive is increased and as a result the concentration of the contraceptive in the patient's blood falls. Because of this fall in concentration, the contraceptive fails to work effectively and the patient is at risk of becoming pregnant.

Being able to identify drugs and other chemicals that increase CYP450 enzyme activity will help to avoid potentially serious drug interactions. The following mnemonic can help you to remember some common enzyme inducers:

Rapid Medicines Management for Healthcare Professionals, First Edition. Paul Deslandes, Simon Young and Ben Pitcher.
© 2020 John Wiley & Sons Ltd. Published 2020 by John Wiley & Sons Ltd.

SCRAP GP

Sulphonylureas (for the treatment of diabetes)
Carbamazepine (for the treatment of seizures, pain, and mood disorders)
Rifampicin (for the treatment of tuberculosis and other infections)
Alcohol
Phenytoin (for the treatment of seizures)
Griseofulvin (for the treatment of fungal infections)
Phenobarbital (for the treatment of seizures)

An important chemical that is not listed in the mnemonic is cigarette smoke. Some of the chemical substances in cigarette smoke are inducers (increase the activity) of the CYP1A2 enzyme and can result in drug interactions.

It has been suggested that not all types of CYP450 enzyme activity can be induced by drugs and other chemicals. For example, the activity of CYP2D6 can vary with a patient's genetic phenotype, but may not be induced significantly by drugs.

Enzyme inhibitors

The proton pump inhibitor esomeprazole is a known CYP450 enzyme inhibitor. Esomeprazole inhibits the activity of CYP2C19 enzymes in the body. The process of inhibition 'prevents' or reduces the metabolic functioning of the enzyme, making it far less efficient at altering the drugs that it metabolises. As a result, the amount of the affected drug in the body can be increased, which may lead to adverse effects or even toxicity.

Example: esomeprazole's effect on the efficacy of phenytoin

Esomeprazole inhibits the activity of CYP2C19, the enzyme that metabolises phenytoin. The enzyme's ability to metabolise the phenytoin is decreased, and as a result the concentration of the phenytoin in the patient's blood rises. Because of this rise in concentration, the patient is at increased risk of adverse effects of the phenytoin such as drowsiness and confusion. Changes in phenytoin levels may be particularly problematic, as this drug has a narrow therapeutic range and small increases in plasma levels can result in risk of toxicity.

Being able to identify drugs and other chemicals that decrease CYP450 enzyme activity will help to avoid potentially serious drug interactions. The following mnemonic can help you to remember some common enzyme inhibitors:

SICKFACES.COM

Sodium valproate (for the treatment of seizures and mood disorders)
Isoniazid (for the treatment of tuberculosis)
Cimetidine (for the treatment of gastro-oesophageal reflux disease and peptic ulcer)
Ketoconazole (for the treatment of fungal infections)
Fluconazole (for the treatment of fungal infections)
Alcohol
Chloramphenicol (for the treatment of bacterial infections)
Erythromycin (for the treatment of bacterial infections)
Sulphonamides (for the treatment of bacterial infections)
Ciprofloxacin (for the treatment of bacterial infections)
Omeprazole (for the treatment of gastro-oesophageal reflux disease and peptic ulcer)
Metronidazole (for the treatment of bacterial infections)

15 Elimination

Drug molecules, whether or not they have undergone metabolic transformation, need to eventually be removed from the body. The process of removal of these compounds from the body is known as elimination (or excretion). Whilst drugs can be eliminated in faeces, hair, sweat, and the water vapour present in the breath, the main route for eliminating drug molecules from the body is in the urine. As the kidneys are the organs that control urine formation, they are the key organs considered when appraising drug elimination.

Drugs can be excreted by the kidney through the following mechanisms:

1. Drugs that are highly water soluble and not bound to plasma proteins will pass into the renal tubule with the glomerular filtrate.
2. Drug molecules that are bound to plasma proteins cannot pass easily through the glomerulus, but may be eliminated via active secretory mechanisms (transporter proteins). Examples include penicillin and morphine. Free drug may also be eliminated by this mechanism.

Why are water-soluble drugs more easily eliminated via the kidney?

As the glomerular filtrate travels through the nephron, water is reabsorbed and the filtrate becomes more concentrated. In the renal tubule, more water is reabsorbed and any drug present in the filtrate will be at a higher concentration than in the surrounding tissue. As a result, if the drug is lipid soluble it will move by passive diffusion out of the filtrate, across the surrounding cell membranes, and into the surrounding tissues, preventing it from being eliminated. In contrast, more water-soluble drugs, which are less able to pass through the membranes of the surrounding epithelial cells, remain in the filtrate (despite the concentration gradient). These drugs are therefore more easily eliminated via the kidney in the urine.

The importance of renal (kidney) function

Because the kidneys are responsible for eliminating many drugs from the body, renal (kidney) function is an important consideration in medication selection and use. If the kidneys cannot facilitate the elimination of a given drug (e.g. due to a disease process that results in reduced renal function), then the drug and any metabolites may accumulate in the body. This increased amount of the drug (and where applicable its metabolites) in the body may result in additional adverse effects or toxicity.

When managing a medicine, whether at the phase of initiation, during its ongoing use, or during withdrawal of the therapy, renal function may need to be monitored. Poor renal function, a deterioration in renal function or kidney injury may necessitate dosage adjustment or even a change in the medication prescribed. Dosage adjustment can be achieved by changing the frequency of drug administration or the amount of drug administered at each dose.

Rapid Medicines Management for Healthcare Professionals, First Edition. Paul Deslandes, Simon Young and Ben Pitcher.
© 2020 John Wiley & Sons Ltd. Published 2020 by John Wiley & Sons Ltd.

The *British National Formulary* (BNF), standard medical texts, and biochemistry departments use universally recognised and validated tools to estimate renal function in order to support medicine management decisions. The most common methods for estimating renal function are the estimated glomerular filtration rate (eGFR) and estimated creatinine clearance. The BNF and other texts provide detailed guidance on the use of equations to calculate these measures. Necessary dosage adjustments based upon these measures can be found in the BNF or the Summary of Product Characteristics (SmPC) for the medicine. Consideration of age, gender, extremes of muscle mass, and diet may need to be made when estimating renal function.

Clinical pharmacological considerations

When medication is used in renal impairment, accumulation of toxic parent drug and/or metabolites is not the only concern. The patient may become more sensitive to the effects of certain drugs even if the elimination of the drugs appears to be unimpaired. Sensitivity to, and tolerance of, side effects may be modified in those with renal impairment. Some drugs require appropriate renal function in order to exert their actions. Many drugs have nephrotoxic properties and their use should be carefully considered in all patients, especially those with existing renal impairment.

Biliary excretion and enterohepatic recycling

Some drugs will be transported into the gall bladder through an active secretory mechanism (transporter protein) in the liver. The drug will then be secreted into the gastrointestinal tract with the bile and eliminated in the faeces. This may be the main route of elimination for the drug, or the drug may be eliminated via a combination of this and other routes (typically the kidney).

For certain drugs, once they are in the intestine a process of reabsorption occurs, resulting in the drug being delivered back into the body. The drug then passes through the liver and into the bile again, repeating the cycle. This process is known as enterohepatic recycling. The drug is typically eliminated after several cycles through the liver and by renal elimination.

Elimination half-life

An important factor to consider when dosing medicines is the elimination half-life. This is the time taken for the plasma concentration of the drug to reduce by half. The half-life can be used to indicate how long it will take for a drug to be removed from the body after treatment discontinuation. The concentration of a drug typically falls below the therapeutic range five half-lives after discontinuation, and 99% of the drug will be eliminated after seven half-lives.

The half-life of different drugs can vary from a matter of a few minutes (e.g. for the inotrope dobutamine) to several days (e.g. the benzodiazepine diazepam). Drugs with a very short half-life must be given by continuous infusion if a consistent plasma level is required, whereas drugs with a longer half-life can be dosed less frequently. For example, a drug with a 24 hour half-life will typically be dosed on a once a day basis.

SECTION II

Applied Theory

16 Routes of Administration: Oral

Administration via the oral route typically involves the patient swallowing the medicine, with subsequent absorption of the drug from the gastrointestinal tract, typically the small intestine. Oral administration is the most commonly used means of administering medications. Administration via the gastrointestinal tract is sometimes termed 'enteral administration', although it can be unclear whether this term also includes the rectal route.

The purpose of the gastrointestinal system is to facilitate the internalisation of external substances into the body. The small intestine has a large surface area designed to maximise absorption of substances the body needs and it is easy to take advantage of this to achieve the internalisation (absorption) of orally administered drugs. As this process is quite natural to people, most patients find swallowing tablets and other oral dose forms convenient and less painful than other routes of administration.

Many (but not all) drugs can be absorbed via the gastrointestinal tract and are suitable for oral administration. For patients with nasogastric (NG) and other feeding tubes in place, some drugs can be administered via these tubes with absorption via the gastrointestinal tract.

The oral route permits a surprising diversity of dosage forms (see below) that have their own advantages and disadvantages, but which can generally be tailored to the requirements of individual patients.

Oral dose formulations

Tablets are the default solid dosage form of oral medicines. Typically, they comprise a specific standardised quantity of the active ingredient along with an inactive bulking agent such as lactose. Whilst some tablets are uncoated others are provided with a coating, which may be intended to make them more palatable or to protect them from the acid environment of the stomach.

Capsules are small two-part containers filled with the drug (usually in the form of a powder). The capsule shell is typically made of gelatine (made from animal bones). This can sometimes cause difficulties for patients who do not wish to consume animal products (e.g. vegans) or who do not wish to consume the products of specific animals (Muslims may wish to avoid pork gelatine and Hindus may wish to avoid bovine gelatine). Alternate dosage forms may be required in these circumstances.

Modified-release tablets or capsules

A modified-release oral medication is a preparation designed to allow the gradual absorption of the drug dose over an extended period of time. This is useful for drugs that have a short half-life where a normal release preparation would require multiple doses throughout

Rapid Medicines Management for Healthcare Professionals, First Edition. Paul Deslandes, Simon Young and Ben Pitcher.
© 2020 John Wiley & Sons Ltd. Published 2020 by John Wiley & Sons Ltd.

the day. A modified-release preparation typically only requires one or two daily doses depending upon the specific formulation. This is of course preferential for patients and can help to improve concordance with a treatment plan.

Modified release is often abbreviated to MR but tablets or capsules may also be denoted with an *ER*, *SR*, *XR* or *XL* suffix (for extended release, sustained release, extended release and extended release, respectively). The individual medications often have features in their name that give an indication of their modified-release nature (e.g. Epilim Chrono®, Tildiem Retard®). Within the *British National Formulary* a modified-release preparation is signified by 'm/r'.

Oral liquids

Tablets and capsules are generally well tolerated and can be easily swallowed by most people. However, young children and adults with swallowing difficulties may not be able to swallow these solid dosage forms. A liquid formulation may be used instead.

Oral liquid preparations may be syrups, suspensions, or dissolvable tablets. These are generally easier to swallow than tablets or capsules, and can be administered via feeding tubes such as NG tubes if required.

Crushing tablets

Whilst many medicines are available in liquid form, not all are (or they may not be available in all care environments). This poses a problem: how do you administer a tablet to patient who cannot swallow a tablet? One of the most common solutions is to crush the tablet. While this may be necessary (and is widely undertaken) it is important to acknowledge the significance of what is being undertaken. By crushing the tablet, the practitioner is changing the formulation, creating an unlicensed medication or is at least using it against the manufacturer's instruction ('off-label'). This is not prohibited, but should not be undertaken lightly. It should generally be discussed with the prescriber or pharmacist and should be discussed with the patient to ensure that they give consent for the off-label use of the medicine.

It is also important to consider how crushing the tablet may affect the proper function of the drug. It has been discussed above that some oral preparations may have a protective coating or may be formulated in a way to facilitate a slow release. Crushing these tablets will disrupt their normal functioning and could either render them ineffective. Alternatively, it may lead to an effective overdose by releasing the dose all at once when it was intended to be released gradually over the course of a day.

Disadvantages

Whilst the oral route may be convenient and suitable for a large number of drugs, it is not perfect. There are reasons why it cannot be used in every situation.

If the chemical nature of a drug means that it is not absorbed effectively across the walls of the gastrointestinal tract or is destroyed by stomach acid or digestive enzymes, then the oral route will not be appropriate. Similarly, even if a drug is absorbed across the intestinal wall, it will be absorbed into the hepatic portal vein. This will carry the drug to the liver, where it may be metabolised before it is able to enter the systemic blood supply in a process called first-pass metabolism. As discussed in Chapter 11, bioavailability describes the proportion of the administered drug that reaches the systemic blood supply. Due to first-pass metabolism, the bioavailability of drugs administered orally is usually significantly lower than when the same drug is administered intravenously.

The proportion of drug that is absorbed may be significantly affected by the presence of food in the stomach. This may require the drug to be administered either before or after food. This can sometimes be represented on a prescription or drug chart with the abbreviation a.c. (short for *ante cibum*) meaning 'before food' or p.c. (short for *post cibum*) meaning 'after food'.

Whilst there are exceptions, drugs administered via the oral route can have a slow onset of action. Although this is not a problem for an ongoing regular medication, it is a limitation if the medication is required to provide rapid relief from symptoms such as severe pain. In such circumstances, other routes such as intravenous or inhalation can give near instantaneous relief.

17 Routes of Administration: Inhalation

The inhalation route of administration refers to the delivery of drugs via the lungs. Typically, the patient breathes in through some form of delivery device and the inspiratory effort carries the drug particles into the lungs.

Local and systemic effects

Drugs delivered via the inhaled route may be intended to act locally on the airways and lungs. Alternatively, they may be intended to be absorbed through the alveoli and into the systemic circulation.

Drugs intended to act locally are generally associated with the treatment of respiratory diseases such as asthma or chronic obstructive pulmonary disease. These include bronchodilators and inhaled corticosteroids.

Drugs intended to act systemically are most commonly associated with analgesia (such as Entonox®) or anaesthesia (sevoflurane), although other drugs acting on the central nervous system, such as nicotine and the antipsychotic loxapine, have also been formulated for delivery via the lung.

Advantages and disadvantages

For drugs acting locally in the airways and lung, inhalational delivery allows the drug to access the site of action without the need for systemic absorption. This reduces the impact of first-pass metabolism and a smaller dose can be administered, with the potential to reduce adverse effects. However, it must be noted that there will nevertheless be some systemic absorption of drugs intended to act locally, with resulting adverse effects on other body systems.

A disadvantage of this route is the need for the use of delivery devices (see below) to administer the drug. These can be difficult for patients to use and may lead to problems with concordance.

Delivery devices

There is a huge range of inhaler devices available, associated with different manufacturers and different medicines such as bronchodilators and inhaled corticosteroids. Each device requires a different technique for optimal use, and therefore has advantages and disadvantages. Tailoring the device to the patient is important to maximise effectiveness. These different devices are described by specific terminology.

Rapid Medicines Management for Healthcare Professionals, First Edition. Paul Deslandes, Simon Young and Ben Pitcher.
© 2020 John Wiley & Sons Ltd. Published 2020 by John Wiley & Sons Ltd.

MDI *(metered dose inhaler)*. The non-specific term for an inhaler that delivers a given dose of drug to be inhaled. This is in contrast to a nebuliser, which produces a continuous flow of nebulised drug for the patient to inhale.

pMDI *(pressurised metered dose inhaler)*. This is the commonly seen inhaler centred around a small canister inside a small pipe-shaped device. This device is typically actuated by pressing downwards on the cylinder, resulting in the delivery of the drug as an aerosol. The actuation of the device needs to be timed with inhalation or the drug will not be delivered properly into the lung. Some devices are available that do not require co-ordination of actuation and breathing (e.g. Easi-breathe®).

DPI *(dry powder inhaler)*. Unlike a pMDI where the drug is stored in a pressurised cylinder and delivered as an aerosol, the DPI delivers individually packaged quantities of powdered drug.

Spacer. A spacer is barrel-shaped chamber (which looks like an empty water bottle). A pMDI is connected to one end and the other end is placed into the patient's mouth. The pMDI is actuated to fill the chamber with the dose of aerosolized drug. The patient can then breath in and out, delivering the drug to the lungs without having to co-ordinate their breathing or holding their breath. It is important that the spacer is compatible with the inhaler as not all pMDIs fit all spacers.

Nebuliser. Whilst hand-held delivery devices are the norm for long-term control of chronic respiratory diseases, when a patient is admitted to hospital with an acute deterioration of respiratory function, a nebuliser may be used to deliver a larger amount of drug to the lungs. A nebuliser consists of a mask with a drug receptacle (chamber) attached to the front. A liquid form of the drug is placed in the chamber and oxygen (or air) is blown through the chamber, vaporising (or nebulising) it. The patient is then able to inhale a continuous flow of drug via the mask.

For most patients who require respiratory drugs to be delivered in this way, additional oxygen is usually required or at least useful. Therefore, nebulisation of the drug is achieved by attaching the tubing to an oxygen supply (such as the oxygen port in a hospital bed area or a canister of medical oxygen). However, it is important to remember that this may be problematic for patients with type 2 respiratory depression and may result in CO_2 retention. In this case, it is necessary to use air rather than medical oxygen to achieve the nebulisation of the drug. This is often done by using a form of compressor, an electric motorised pump to deliver the flow of air to the nebuliser mask.

Particle size

Delivery of drug via the inhaled route relies upon the drug being in powder form or rendered in an airborne droplet form that can be inhaled. The drug particle size that is produced by the device affects how and where the drug is deposited in the airways and lung. This can mean that different inhalation devices that produce different sized particles can require different dosages of the same drug to achieve the same effect. An example of this is the Clenil® and QVAR® beclometasone inhalers, which have differing potencies at the same microgram dose.

Inhaler technique

The effectiveness of a drug delivered via the inhaled route is dependent upon how much of the dose reaches the lungs. When using a form of hand-held delivery device this is highly dependent on inhaler technique. Whilst the use of an inhaler seems to be straightforward and appears to be simply a matter of 'sticking it in your mouth and sucking', it can be difficult to do correctly. Some of the most common difficulties stem from the challenge presented by synchronising the actuation of the device (pressing the button) and inhaling. The result of poor inhaler technique is that the drug is either immediately exhaled or is deposited in the throat rather than the lungs. If the drug is deposited in the throat it will be swallowed. While this may allow the drug to be absorbed via the gastrointestinal tract, its effect will be reduced and its onset of action slower.

Poor inhaler technique is such a widespread problem that if a given treatment regime appears to be ineffective, the first thing to do is check the patient's technique. The specifics of correct inhaler technique will vary from device to device and from drug to drug. It is important to check the appropriate instructions provided by the manufacturer or supplied by your place of work to ensure that your patient is using the correct technique. pMDIs are particularly associated with poor inhaler technique, and various strategies have been developed to improve this. One of these is the use of a spacer (as described above), which has proved to be significantly more effective at delivering drug into the lung.

Inspiratory effort

Some inhalation devices (especially dry powder inhalers such as the Turbohaler® used in Symbicort®) require a significant inspiratory effort to deliver the drug particles to the lungs. This is a limitation, as the drug is by definition prescribed to people who have respiratory disease and therefore may well have reduced respiratory function. A patient's inspiratory flow rate is typically measured by the doctor before the device is prescribed. However, the inspiratory flow rate may be reduced during an exacerbation of their respiratory disease, which could result in the treatment being less effective.

18 Routes of Administration: Topical

Topical administration describes the application of a drug directly onto the surface of the tissue that requires the treatment. The most obvious examples of drugs administered this way are creams and ointments applied directly to the skin. However, other routes such as inhalation and intranasal can be considered topical when the drug is being used to treat the surface of the lung (e.g. salbutamol) or nasal cavity (e.g. mometasone), respectively. This provides the benefits of systemic administration, but typically at a lower dose and with reduced potential for adverse effects. However, these methods are generally referred to as 'inhaled' and 'intranasal' whilst 'topical' is generally taken to mean creams, ointments, lotions, or eye drops.

Advantages

One of the main advantages of using a topical route of administration is the ability to apply the drug to the precise area of the body that needs it. If a patient has a diseased area of skin, it is possible to treat it systemically via the oral route. However, when dosing the drug orally, it must pass through and be absorbed by the digestive system and then the liver before being dispersed throughout the entire bloodstream and finally diffusing through the tissues to the skin itself. It is necessary to give a significant quantity of the drug via this route in order to achieve effective concentrations in the skin. This also means that the drug could potentially affect tissues throughout the entire body, significantly increasing the chance and severity of adverse effects.

In contrast, topical administration of the same drug requires a tiny fraction of the dose to be directly applied to the affected area. In this case, it does not have to pass through the digestive system nor disperse through the tissues, so may act more quickly. Furthermore, because the drug is applied directly to the required site of action, its adverse effects are more likely to be local rather than systemic. Whilst it is possible for the drug to be absorbed through the skin and enter the general circulation resulting in systemic adverse effects, if these do occur they are likely to be milder than if the drug was administered systemically. For example, patients with eczema benefit from the use of steroids. An oral steroid (e.g. prednisolone) will be effective in reducing this inflammatory skin condition, but may lead to significant systemic adverse effects (such as adrenal suppression, fluid retention, nausea, and osteoporosis). In contrast, a steroid cream (e.g. hydrocortisone) will be similarly effective but with adverse effects more likely to be limited to local reactions rather than systemic effects.

It is worth noting that a contraindication to a drug due to a systemic side effect may still apply even if the drug is being used topically. Ibuprofen is typically contraindicated in patients with a history of gastric ulcers. The use of topical ibuprofen gel may seem like a good option for treating a painful joint to achieve a localised anti-inflammatory effect

Rapid Medicines Management for Healthcare Professionals, First Edition. Paul Deslandes, Simon Young and Ben Pitcher.
© 2020 John Wiley & Sons Ltd. Published 2020 by John Wiley & Sons Ltd.

without the systemic adverse effects. However, manufacturers of ibuprofen gel may still advise that it should not be used in patients with a history of gastric ulcers due to the risk of absorption through the skin and an increased risk of gastrointestinal bleeding.

Dosing and application considerations

Whilst a specific topical cream or ointment may be available in different strengths, there is still the question of how much to apply. Whilst some medications provide instructions such as 'use sparingly' this may not give a clear indication of how much to apply. One option describing the dosing of creams and ointments that is used in some areas is the fingertip unit (FTU).

An FTU is a measure defined as the amount of cream squeezed from a tube onto a finger, from the tip to the fold of the first knuckle. A patient can therefore be given instructions of how many FTUs should be applied to a given body part (typically one FTU is enough to cover an area twice the size of an adult's hand). Whilst variations in hand size make this far from an exact measure, it provides a useful, pragmatic guide for practitioners and patients alike.

Eye drops

Eye drops are a form of topical liquid dose formulation where a drug is dropped into an open eye from a small bottle. This can be difficult for some patients due to co-morbid illness such as arthritis or Parkinson's disease, which make manipulation of a small container difficult. Devices are available to facilitate the use of eyedrop bottles and may help in these circumstances. It can also be difficult to prevent blinking, which may deflect the drug from the eye.

Dosing is usually described in terms of number of drops into each eye, but this can be quite inexact. The eye can typically only hold one drop of liquid applied at a time, and any more than this tends to immediately run out of the eye. When administering eye drops (especially those used to treat infection such as chloramphenicol), it is often recommended that a separate eyedrop container be used for each eye to avoid cross-infection.

As with other routes of topical administration, it is important to remember that drugs applied to the eye may result in systemic adverse effects. An example is the use of non-selective beta-blocker eye drops (e.g. timolol), which may result in bronchoconstriction, a particular problem in asthmatic patients.

Disadvantages of topical administration

As mentioned above, one of the main disadvantages of topical administration, particularly to the eye or airways, is the difficulty of using administration devices. Inhaler devices designed to deliver drugs to the airways are particularly difficult to use (see also Chapter 17), whilst administering medicines to the eye may be particularly stressful for small children.

Although topical administration can help to reduce the required dose of a drug and its associated adverse effects, both local and systemic unwanted effects can still occur. Patients may also be sensitive to the excipients used in the formulation of creams and ointments, resulting in allergic reactions at the site of application.

19 Routes of Administration: Transdermal

The transdermal route and its dosage forms deliver drugs across the skin to achieve systemic distribution of the drug. The most commonly encountered transdermal dosage form is the transdermal patch. Transdermal semi-solid formulations such as gels are also used.

Transdermal patches

Transdermal patches are sophisticated medical plasters. They typically contain a reservoir of the drug, which is delivered gradually over time. Patches are particularly useful and are most frequently utilised when a controlled release of medication may be advantageous over a period of many hours (typically 12–72 hours but sometimes longer). The first patch used in the UK contained the drug scopolamine, which is licenced for the prevention of travel sickness symptoms (Scopoderm®).

The skin functions as an efficient barrier to protect the body and as a consequence only certain medications with particular physico-chemical properties are suitable for transdermal delivery. One of the most frequently encountered patches is the nicotine patch. Nicotine can be relatively easily delivered across the skin and the patch acts as an ideal dosage form for the controlled release of the nicotine. The steady release of nicotine through the skin to the bloodstream forms an ideal means of staving off the craving to smoke a cigarette. Other commonly encountered formulations include the administration of the opioid medications buprenorphine and fentanyl to provide a continuous delivery of analgesic. Patches containing female sex hormones such as oestrogen are used for contraceptive and hormone placement/replacement purposes. Other medications that are delivered via patches include rivastigmine for the treatment of Alzheimer's disease and rotigotine for Parkinson's disease.

One way to overcome the barrier to drug delivery presented by the skin is the use of microneedle technology. This approach uses ultra-fine needles to facilitate the transfer of drugs across the skin whose properties would not normally allow transdermal delivery. This is likely to be increasingly adopted as a delivery mechanism in the future.

Considerations when using patches

- Patches should be placed on dry skin.
- Oils, lotions, and other cosmetics should not be present in or on the skin when the patch is placed.
- Patches should be placed on a hairless (non-hairy) area of the body.
- Sites of application should be rotated in order to avoid skin irritation.
- The skin at the site of application should not be broken, irritated, or irradiated.
- The patch needs to be placed on a flat surface – usually on the torso or the upper arm.

Rapid Medicines Management for Healthcare Professionals, First Edition. Paul Deslandes, Simon Young and Ben Pitcher.
© 2020 John Wiley & Sons Ltd. Published 2020 by John Wiley & Sons Ltd.

- Patches should be inspected with care before placement – damaged patches can alter the release characteristics of the medication.
- Patches should be applied immediately after being removed from the packaging.
- Patches should be worn for their licensed period of use and then removed and replaced (unless a discontinuation protocol has been put in place).
- Patients who have suffered adverse events as a result of patch use (and have had the patch removed and its further use discontinued) should be monitored for suitable periods of time after the patch has been removed as the effects of the drug can continue for a significant period after patch removal.
- Care should be taken to ensure that patches do not stick to another person. This is especially important with strong opioids such as fentanyl.
- Direct heat such as saunas, sunbeds, electric blankets, etc. can alter the release characteristic of the formulations and expose the patient to adverse effects. This is a very important consideration in the case of the strong opioids.

Advantages and disadvantages

Transdermal delivery allows administration of a drug over an extended period without the need for repeated dosing. This can be more convenient for the patient and is also useful where other routes are not appropriate (e.g. patients with swallowing difficulties). The continuous release of the drug from the patch also reduces the peaks and troughs in drug plasma levels that may be associated with other formulations.

Whilst the gradual release of the drug from the patch helps to maintain a steady plasma concentration over time, it can result in a delay in the onset of action. As a result, transdermal delivery via patches may not be suitable for the management of unstable conditions (e.g. acute pain). Care should be taken to avoid contact with a discarded patch. When a patch is removed, the reservoir will still contain some of the drug and safe disposal of the patch is important to avoid accidental administration to anyone handling it.

20 Routes of Administration: Injection

Whilst the enteral route is suitable for the administration of many medicines and is commonly used, it may at times be unusable due to nausea and vomiting or swallowing difficulties, or it may be ineffective for a given drug such as insulin. In these instances, an alternative route must be used. One option is to deliver drugs directly into a specific tissue via injection or cannula, literally inserting a needle or cannula through the skin and delivering the drug into the tissue. The most common forms of injection are intravenous, intramuscular, and subcutaneous.

Intravenous

The intravenous route (often abbreviated to i/v) describes the administration of the drug directly into the blood via a vein. The intravenous route is generally used when it is necessary to get a drug into a patient quickly and reliably (typically in more urgent or serious situations) when other routes are either too slow, result in inconsistent absorption, or are unavailable.

How is it administered?

The i/v route is often thought of in terms of injection using a syringe and needle, however whilst it is certainly possible to inject a drug in this way, it is not done very commonly in health care. Far more commonly a patient will have a peripheral venous cannula inserted. This is a thin tube inserted into the vein with a port to which a syringe or infusion line can be attached with relative ease. This allows medicines to be delivered i/v without having to locate and penetrate a vein with a needle every time they are administered.

A venous cannula can be described in a variety of different ways, including:

- 'having a line inserted'
- 'i/v access'
- 'Venflon®' which is a brand name for a cannula that is widely used.

Bolus or infusion?

Medicines can be administered intravenously either as a bolus (a single measure of a drug administered via syringe) or as a continuous infusion. As discussed above, syringes with needles are rarely used to deliver drugs via the i/v route, instead the syringe is attached to an access port on the venous cannula. Continuous infusion involves adding a drug to a bag of fluid (e.g. normal saline) which is then administered using either gravity or an electrically powered pump to cause the fluid to flow into the patient through plastic tubing, often called a 'giving set'.

Rapid Medicines Management for Healthcare Professionals, First Edition. Paul Deslandes, Simon Young and Ben Pitcher.
© 2020 John Wiley & Sons Ltd. Published 2020 by John Wiley & Sons Ltd.

Before administering a medicine via a venous cannula it is usually necessary to 'flush' the line with a small quantity of normal saline to make sure that the catheter is patent. This is typically repeated after the medicine has been administered to make sure that there is no residue left in the cannula.

Whilst many medicines given i/v may be available in liquid form (often in a glass ampoule), some are stored in powder form. These must typically be reconstituted with specific quantities of normal saline or water for injection prior to administration. The specifics of how to reconstitute these medicines can typically be found in the information leaflet supplied with the medication.

Due to the additional risks associated with administration via the i/v route, staff are required to be specifically trained or qualified. Most employers and healthcare providers require practitioners to undergo additional training and demonstrate competence before they are allowed to administer medicines i/v. This usually includes additional numeracy assessments to ensure the practitioner is capable of the necessary drug calculations. It is also standard practice to undertake two checks of all medicines to be administered i/v to ensure that they are correct and safe.

Advantages of the i/v route

As administration is directly into the bloodstream, it bypasses many of the potential barriers that can affect a drug's speed and completeness of absorption. Additionally, as the drug enters the venous bloodstream it is carried directly to heart, allowing it to be readily dispersed throughout the entire blood volume.

Veins are relatively insensitive, meaning that generally they are not adversely affected by most drugs administered into them. However, some drugs can be more irritant than others and may result in loss of the access point.

Disadvantages of the i/v route

Pharmacokinetics

The fact that drugs enter the blood quickly via the i/v route is a double-edged sword. Whilst this can allow the drug to act quickly, it also increases the potential for the concentration of the drug in the body to rise so quickly that it reaches toxic levels. To avoid this, i/v administration is done in a measured way, typically at a rate of 1 ml per minute or slower. It is important to bear this in mind when preparing to administer a drug via this route in order to allocate an appropriate amount of time and position yourself appropriately to allow you to accomplish this safely and comfortably.

Risk of infection

By puncturing the skin of a patient, injections circumvent the protection from infection that the skin provides. Because of this, use of i/v administration leads to a higher risk of infection than other routes. For this reason, all equipment (syringes, giving sets) and the medicines themselves must be sterile. This adds to the cost of manufacture and complexity of preparation.

Extravasation

If a peripheral venous cannula is disrupted, it can result in the infusion being deposited into the tissues surrounding the vein rather than into the vein itself. This is called 'extravasation', although it is frequently referred to as having 'tissued'. If the drug enters the tissue in this way it will be at concentrations far higher than intended and can cause adverse effects.

Due to the potential for infection or extravasation, it is important that if a venous catheter is in situ it is visually inspected on a regular basis. This is sometimes problematic if the venous catheter is covered with a dressing or bandage (often in an attempt to prevent it from being dislodged).

Subcutaneous injection

Drugs can be injected into the layer of subcutaneous fat found between the skin and the muscle. This method of subcutaneous injection is often abbreviated to 'sub cut' or SC. This route can be used to achieve a localised effect in the specific tissue (e.g. local anaesthetic) or with the expectation that the drug will be absorbed into the blood supply for a systemic effect (e.g. insulin).

How is it administered?

If the drug is not being administered into a specific tissue, then it is typically injected into the lower abdomen (around the umbilicus), the upper arm or the thigh. A syringe and needle or prefilled device (such as a pen device containing a small vial of the drug) are typically used. Unlike intramuscular or intravenous administration, subcutaneous administration requires minimal training and has less risk of accidental harm. As such, patients are frequently able to self-administer via this route.

Advantages of the subcutaneous route

Injecting the drug into the subcutaneous fat does achieve a high bioavailability, although the absorption of the drug into the blood supply takes time. This produces a slower onset of action than intravenous injection, but therefore provides a more sustained duration of effect and reduces the potential for toxicity.

Disadvantages of the subcutaneous route

One-off dosing of a drug via the subcutaneous route has few disadvantages (aside from the discomfort of the injection itself). However, when it is used on a longer-term basis with repeated regular injections (such as for enoxaparin or insulin) there is significant potential for pain, irritation or other side effects at the site of injection. This can in some cases be ameliorated by rotating the site of injection.

Intramuscular injection

The intramuscular route is generally used less commonly than the intravenous, or subcutaneous routes. However, for certain drugs it has useful properties. Intramuscular injections (often abbreviated to i/m) are typically administered using a standard syringe and needle, although some medicines are produced in a specific delivery device.

Advantages of the intramuscular route

When a medicine is injected into the muscle, it is possible to deposit a reservoir of drug into the tissue that will be absorbed over an extended period of time. This provides maintenance drug concentrations without the need for frequent repeated dosing and is more convenient for the patient. Use of this route can also help to reduce unintentional non-concordance with treatment, as the patient does not have to remember to take the medication on a daily basis.

Disadvantages of the intramuscular route

To inject into the muscle, the needle must be inserted though many layers of tissue. It is therefore important to ensure that the needle used is long enough to reach the muscle. If the needle is not inserted correctly, there is significant potential for it to damage nerves, bone or blood vessels. The accidental insertion of the needle into a blood vessel carries the additional risk of unintentionally administering the drug intravenously and essentially overdosing the patient. Due to these potential risks the administration of intramuscular injections is typically only undertaken by trained staff.

21 Routes of Administration: Rectal

The rectal route of administration can be used to deliver medicines locally to the rectum or colon, or to the systemic circulation. This route of administration may be useful when a medicine is unstable in the acid environment of the stomach or in patients unable to swallow. A number of different formulations are available to administer medicines rectally, and research is ongoing to further develop this aspect of drug delivery.

Absorption from the rectum

There are a number of differences when a medicine is administered via the rectum rather than orally to the upper gastrointestinal tract. A key factor is the avoidance of the stomach, and its associated acid conditions and digestive enzymes. The rectum has a pH of around 7 and does not exhibit significant enzymatic activity. As a result, drugs are less readily degraded in the rectum, which may improve bioavailability. Drugs acting on the central nervous system are well suited to rectal administration as they must be lipid soluble to cross the blood–brain barrier and this also helps to facilitate rectal absorption. Rectally administered formulations of opioid analgesics, benzodiazepines, and the antiepileptic carbamazepine are all available in the UK.

The rectum is supplied by a number of different blood vessels, some of which take blood to the liver, resulting in first-pass metabolism. Other vessels avoid the liver, and drugs absorbed through these will bypass first-pass metabolism. An absence of cytochrome P450 activity in the rectum compared with the intestinal wall also reduces first-pass effects, all of which may help to increase bioavailability. However, drug absorption from the rectum is influenced by other factors such as pH, fluid volume, motility, and rectal contents, and can therefore be somewhat variable.

What formulations are given rectally?

Drugs administered rectally are typically formulated as either suppositories or enemas for systemic or local effects, or creams or ointments for local effects.

Suppositories are solid dosage forms that release the drug as they melt in the rectum. They can be used to achieve systemic effects (such as certain non-steroidal anti-inflammatory drugs or morphine for analgesia) or local effects (such as glycerine for constipation). Rectal creams and ointments can be used for a local action, for example corticosteroids and local anaesthetics to reduce pain and inflammation associated with haemorrhoids, or glyceryl trinitrate for the treatment of anal fissure. Enemas are liquid medicine preparations, often used for their effects on the colon and rectum. Phosphate enemas are used for bowel evacuation prior to certain procedures. Mesalazine is an anti-inflammatory used in the treatment of ulcerative colitis of the distal colon and rectum. When administered as a rectal

Rapid Medicines Management for Healthcare Professionals, First Edition. Paul Deslandes, Simon Young and Ben Pitcher.
© 2020 John Wiley & Sons Ltd. Published 2020 by John Wiley & Sons Ltd.

enema it combines some local and systemic effects. Diazepam is an example of a medicine that is formulated as an enema that has a systemic effect. It is well absorbed from the rectum and is sometimes used in the acute management of seizures.

What are the advantages and disadvantages of rectal administration?

The rectal route of administration is a useful alternative when it is not possible to give drugs to a patient orally. This might be due to nausea and vomiting, lack of consciousness (e.g. post-surgery or associated with an acute illness), or patients with swallowing difficulties (such as the elderly or children). As mentioned above, rectal administration may help to avoid first-pass metabolism and enzymatic degradation of medicines in the stomach, resulting in improved bioavailability. Administration for a local effect may help to reduce systemic exposure to a medicine and reduce associated systemic adverse effects.

A disadvantage of rectal administration is the potential variability in drug absorption, with resulting unpredictability of plasma levels and therapeutic response. Whilst a reduction in gastric irritation is sometimes considered an advantage of the rectal route, the result may be to simply alter the site of irritation. Rectal irritation has been reported following both short- and longer-term use of this route of administration. Another potentially significant disadvantage is a lack of patient acceptability. This may be driven by a number of factors, including social and cultural preconceptions. Given the importance of patient concordance with medication to achieve optimal outcome, any factor likely to affect this requires careful consideration.

22 Drugs in Pregnancy

Drugs that are used in practice, and those that are misused, are xenochemicals (chemicals that are foreign to the body) and the body will attempt to metabolise and eliminate them. This process takes on particular significance in pre-conception, conception, and pregnancy. Drugs taken by the mother/pregnant woman may present a risk to the foetus during the different stages of pregnancy. The nature of the risk varies according to the trimester. The risk of teratogenesis (developmental abnormalities) is highest during the first trimester, whilst foetal growth can be affected later in the pregnancy. Acute effects on the newborn, such as intoxication or withdrawal effects, can be associated with drugs used prior to and during delivery.

A general principle when prescribing drugs in pregnancy is to use the lowest possible dose for the shortest possible duration in order to minimise exposure to the foetus. Specialist advice concerning the use of drugs during pregnancy should be sought from relevant experts such as medicines information support services or the UK Teratology Information service.

Drugs and pre-conception

Drugs can adversely influence the outcomes of pregnancy even before conception takes place. The use of drugs by men or women prior to conception can have an effect on both the likelihood of becoming pregnant and subsequent foetal development. The effects of drugs on fertility has historically focussed on women. However, there is evidence to suggest that drug groups such as anti-depressants, calcium channel blockers, anti-epileptics, and anti-retrovirals can alter the composition of semen and can influence male fertility.

For certain drugs, the provision of adequate contraception forms part of the product licence. Examples include thalidomide and lenalidomide used in the treatment of myeloma, and the anti-epileptic valproate. In April 2018, the Medicines and Healthcare Products Regulatory Agency changed its regulatory position on medicines containing valproate. It advises that if a woman of childbearing age is to be prescribed valproate, she must be enrolled in a pregnancy prevention programme. This is the result of the established link between valproate and teratogenic effects and developmental disorders.

Drugs in pregnancy

It has been established that medicines used by women at all stages of pregnancy have the potential to influence the outcome of that pregnancy. Medicines can affect the development of the foetus during pregnancy, as well as delivery and subsequent development though childhood.

Rapid Medicines Management for Healthcare Professionals, First Edition. Paul Deslandes, Simon Young and Ben Pitcher.
© 2020 John Wiley & Sons Ltd. Published 2020 by John Wiley & Sons Ltd.

Medication should generally be avoided wherever possible during pregnancy. Any medication that is used in pregnancy should be subjected to patient-centred and objective scrutiny. In certain cases (e.g. the management of chronic conditions), the decisions are more challenging as ongoing treatment may be important for the mother's well-being. Medicines will continue to be used where the benefits to the mother outweigh the risks posed to the developing foetus. In many cases, non-pharmacological interventions may represent a preferable alternative to medication. The use of new medicines and those undergoing increased pharmacovigilance is less suitable in pregnant women. Principles such as using medicines for the shortest time possible and at the lowest therapeutic dose particularly apply when considering medication use in pregnancy.

The first trimester of pregnancy (in particular weeks 3–11) is the period when the foetus is most vulnerable to teratogenic influence. The use of medication that is teratogenic at this stage of pregnancy could lead to foetal malformations. Some examples of teratogenic drugs include (but are not limited to) vitamin A derivatives (e.g. isotretinoin), angiotensin converting enzyme inhibitors, and warfarin. For women with long-term conditions who may become pregnant, considering the risks of different treatments prior to initiation may help to avoid foetal exposure should unexpected pregnancy occur. Similarly, women with conditions such as epilepsy should consider the teratogenic potential of their anti-epileptic medication, and plan their pregnancies in discussion with their physician in order that risks can be minimised. This may involve swapping medication that is associated with teratogenesis to a medication that is less likely to be teratogenic. However, it must be noted that this process may itself have a significant impact on the well-being and activities of daily living of the patient. Therefore, factoring in the possibility of future pregnancy when choosing an initial treatment may be preferable.

Medicines used in the second and third trimester of pregnancy can influence foetal growth and development (e.g. beta-blockers). Medicines used close to or during delivery can result in adverse effects in the neonate. Some examples include opioids (e.g. pethidine), associated with respiratory depression and withdrawal effects, benzodiazepines (e.g. diazepam), associated with floppy baby syndrome (due to muscle relaxation), and beta-blockers (e.g. atenolol), associated with bradycardia and hypotension. The use of medication that may influence labour or affect the birthing process also needs to be considered. Drugs such as non-steroidal anti-inflammatory drugs can delay the onset of or prolong labour.

In addition to possible adverse effects on the foetus, it is also important to consider how the effectiveness of medicines is influenced by the physiological changes that occur during pregnancy. For example, physiological changes can affect pharmacokinetic parameters such as volume of distribution. For some drugs (e.g. certain antidepressants), this may result in the need to alter doses as pregnancy progresses in order to maintain the therapeutic effect.

23 Drugs in Breast-feeding

There are two main issues to consider when giving medication to a breast-feeding mother: will the medication be excreted into the milk and will the medication affect the process of lactation?

Medication is eliminated from the body primarily via the kidneys. Drugs are also eliminated/excreted in water vapour in breath (via the respiratory system), through bile, and also through breast milk. Medication that is eliminated via breast milk can pass into the feeding infant and exert an unwanted and potentially adverse pharmacological effect. A consideration of the possible impact on the infant is therefore important when medicines are prescribed for breast-feeding mothers, or when a medicine is purchased over the counter. A careful evaluation of the risks and benefits is required. Where possible, drug use should be avoided unless there is a clear clinical need.

The evidence base

There is a dearth of evidence on the impact of medication on the breast-feeding infant. The application of scientific method in the form of randomised controlled trials to study the effects of medication in this patient group is an unethical approach. A study cannot be deemed appropriate if there is a potential to cause harm. Therefore, evidence on the effect of medication found in breast milk must come from other sources. These include case reports, observational studies, and prediction of the behaviour of a drug based on its physicochemical and pharmacological properties.

Drugs that are new to the market will typically have more limited evidence to support their use in breast-feeding, and greater caution is therefore required.

Lack of evidence of harm does not equate to evidence of safety, merely a lack of evidence.

Pharmacokinetic considerations

Some drugs will not enter the breast milk and therefore will have no effect on the breast-feeding infant. These tend to be large molecules (such as heparin and insulin). Some will only pass into breast milk in small quantities and these quantities will have minimal or no effect on the breast-feeding infant. However, some drugs will pass into breast milk in quantities large enough to influence the physiology of the infant. Factors such as volume of distribution and protein binding can affect the degree to which drugs are transferred into breast milk.

A drug's duration of action is also important when considering its use in breast-feeding. For drugs with a short half-life, it may be possible to time the administration so that the concentration in breast milk is minimised when the infant is feeding. For drugs with a longer half-life this may not be possible and therefore these drugs may be more likely to be transferred to the infant.

Rapid Medicines Management for Healthcare Professionals, First Edition. Paul Deslandes, Simon Young and Ben Pitcher.
© 2020 John Wiley & Sons Ltd. Published 2020 by John Wiley & Sons Ltd.

Infants with hepatic or renal impairment may demonstrate a more pronounced response to drugs that enter the breast milk than those with normal physiological function. Premature infants may also exhibit similar vulnerabilities.

Pharmacodynamic considerations

The pharmacodynamic properties of the administered drug will determine the nature of effect that is seen in the infant. Medication that causes drowsiness may pass into the infant and affect normal circadian rhythms as well as the ability to suckle if the infant is rendered drowsy by the drug. Drugs that are taken in high doses by mothers may have an influence on the infant that would be difficult to predict if the same drug were to be used in lower or mid-range doses. Drugs that are known to provoke hypersensitivity or allergy may also do so in the infant if the exposure is sufficient to provoke that immunological response.

Effects of drugs on lactation

In addition to the possible adverse effects on the foetus, it should also be noted that drugs may have an effect on lactation. Lactation is mediated in part through the effects of prolactin released from the pituitary gland. Control of prolactin release is inhibited by the action of dopamine at its receptors, therefore drugs that interfere with dopaminergic neurotransmission have the ability to alter prolactin release and ultimately lactation.

Dopamine receptor agonists such as bromocriptine and cabergoline will stimulate dopamine receptors, leading to a reduction in prolactin release and inhibition of lactation. This effect is sometimes exploited therapeutically (e.g. to prevent lactation in women following miscarriage or termination of pregnancy).

Dopamine receptor antagonists such as antipsychotics will block the effect of dopamine on the pituitary gland, leading to an increase in prolactin release. As a result, they may be associated with the adverse effects of gynaecomastia (breast enlargement) and galactorrhoea (milk secretion).

24 Drugs in Children

The field of paediatrics is vast and diverse. Whilst entire textbooks have been written on this subject, this chapter will focus on some of the more notable differences that are apparent in the management of medicines for children.

Is a child just like a small adult?

Whilst the child is a smaller human being, differences between child and adult physiology mean that when considering medicines it is not simply possible to scale everything up and down with weight. The underdeveloped body of the child can have significant differences across all areas of pharmacokinetics (absorption, distribution, metabolism, and elimination), changing the way that we use drugs. These differences become more significant when considering children below the age of two years.

Absorption. The immature gastrointestinal system can affect the absorption of drugs. Differences in a baby's gastric pH, gastric emptying, and speed of gastric transit can result in an increased or decreased rate of absorption of different drugs compared to adults.

Distribution. The ratio of muscle to fat and quantities of extracellular fluid will vary in children of different ages compared to adults. A child's blood–brain barrier can be less effective, allowing easier entry of drugs into the central nervous system. Very young children can also have different levels of plasma proteins, which can affect the levels of protein-bound drugs.

Metabolism and elimination. The major organs involved with metabolism and elimination of drugs (the liver and kidney) may not be fully developed in children and may therefore behave differently than in adult patients. This may manifest as an increased or decreased ability to metabolise a specific drug. For example, the half-life of diazepam is half as long in an infant as it is in an adult, whereas the half-life of theophylline is approximately ten times longer than in an adult.

Can it be difficult to administer medicines to children?

It is understandable that younger children may not be able to rationalise the need to experience some small discomfort to receive necessary medical treatment. Certain routes of administration can therefore prove challenging (such as any form of injection), resulting in fear and avoidance behaviours from the child. This is particularly apparent if the medication is unpleasant or painful, or if good administration technique is required for it to be effective. In some instances, this means alternative routes of administration may be used. For example, a nasal route is used for the seasonal flu vaccine whilst adults receive an injection.

Rapid Medicines Management for Healthcare Professionals, First Edition. Paul Deslandes, Simon Young and Ben Pitcher.
© 2020 John Wiley & Sons Ltd. Published 2020 by John Wiley & Sons Ltd.

Some medications have an unpleasant taste, which can cause children to spit them out or even vomit. This causes problems as it becomes impossible to be sure how much of the drug the child has absorbed.

Using pressurised metered dose inhalers with children can be problematic due to the difficulty for them to co-ordinate the use of the device with breathing. Even using a spacer can prove difficult as young children can find the placing of the spacer on the face unpleasant, which can cause them to vigorously resist.

It may be necessary to hold and support the child to make the administration possible. If this is necessary it should be done with the utmost care and where possible the involvement and agreement of the child's parent or carer.

Can children administer medicines themselves?

This of course depends on the age and capability of the child and must be assessed on a patient-by-patient basis. It is also not uncommon for the child's parents or carers to be involved in the administration of medicines and this is usually solely undertaken by them when a child is at home. It is therefore important to ensure that the parent or carer is instructed in how to administer the medication correctly.

Do children get the same dose of drug as an adult?

Typically (and unsurprisingly) children are given a lower dose of drugs than adults. This is either a standardised reduced dose or the dose will be calculated by body weight of the child. It is interesting to note that whilst the actual dose will of course be lower than that of an adult, the dose per kilogram may actually be higher. Calculating drug doses by weight can sometimes give problematic outcomes, especially when calculating a dose for a large child. It can be possible that the dose by weight calculation actually produces a dose that is in excess of the maximum safe dose for any patient and higher than that which is prescribed for an adult. Similarly, a dose calculated for an obese child may actually be a toxic dose (even if the child is heavier it does not mean the liver and kidneys are necessarily capable of dealing with the dose that the large weight suggests). This has led to the practice of dosing based on the ideal weight for a child of that age rather than the child's actual weight. It is therefore common to see standardised doses for specific age ranges.

Covert administration

As some medications can be unpalatable, children may be unwilling to swallow them. In these cases it may be necessary to disguise or hide the medication in food. This is not ideal and presents potential concerns about deceiving patients, the possibility of the medication reacting in some way with the food it is mixed with, and the possibility that the patient will not consume the full dose. It is acknowledged, however, that this may be in the patient's best interests, but the decision to administer covertly should not be made in isolation.

Do we use the same drugs in children as in adults?

In the majority of cases yes, although commonly with an adjusted dose or formulation. However, there are certain drugs that we cannot routinely use in children. These include common drugs such as aspirin, which if given to children with certain infections can precipitate the potentially fatal Reyes syndrome. Antibiotics such as tetracycline, which deposit in the developing bones and teeth, should also be avoided in children.

Whilst children may be involved in the trials of new treatment regimes, their participation occurs only when essential and is generally limited. This can mean that a drug's use in children may not be fully tested by a drug company and may not form part of its Marketing Authorisation (licence). Therefore, the use of some drugs in children is described as 'unlicensed' or 'off-label'. This should be discussed with the patient or their guardian, and considered in all aspects of their medicines management as the risks and benefits of the treatment may be different to when the drug is used within its Marketing Authorisation.

Checking: two nurse or not two nurse?

Due to the fragile nature of paediatric patients and the non-standard dosing that patients receive, it is critical that medication is rigorously checked. To ensure this, it has previously been considered essential for all medications given to children to be checked by two qualified members of staff. However, recently this strategy has been called into question. It has been suggested that the two-nurse checking procedure is not only resource intensive, but may actually be less safe. Both of the nurses checking can sometimes rely on the other to check it properly, when in truth neither are. A nurse who is solely responsible for checking the drug will check it more closely because they know it is entirely down to them. Whilst this change in strategy has been introduced in some areas it is important to follow your local policy regarding the checking of medications.

Gillick consent

It is generally considered that children under the age of 16 are not able to give consent for medical procedures or medication and therefore consent is granted by their parent or guardian. However, a provision does exist that if a child is deemed to have full understanding of the medical treatment, they may consent to the treatment themselves. In the court case in which this ruling was made, one of the parties was Victoria Gillick. This has resulted in the term 'Gillick competent' being used to describe a child able to consent for themselves.

25 Drugs in Hepatic Impairment

The liver is the primary organ responsible for drug metabolism. In considering the pharmacokinetic processes of absorption, distribution, metabolism, and elimination, it is apparent that in order for drugs to be metabolised appropriately, hepatic function is a key factor. If the function of the liver is impaired by disease processes or other damage (e.g. from the excessive consumption of alcohol), metabolic processes may be disrupted and the final elimination of drug from the body may be impeded.

The liver is a relatively resilient organ and hepatic function has to be severely compromised to adversely influence drug metabolism clinically. Liver functions tests, which are commonly measured biochemical markers, are not good indicators of the ability of the liver to metabolise particular drugs or drug groups. In severe hepatic impairment, plasma albumin falls (hypo-albuminaemia) and this may alter the clinical efficacy and the severity of the side effects of drugs, especially those that are highly protein bound. Deranged biochemical markers, such as elevated plasma bilirubin in adults who drink alcohol, can be indicators of more serious hepatic damage (raised bilirubin can also occur in adults in conditions such as Gilbert's syndrome). Clinical signs of hepatic impairment such as ascites, jaundice, and clinical evidence of hepatic encephalopathy are important markers in the evaluation of drug therapy.

As well as its role in drug metabolism, the liver has many other functions in sustaining homeostasis. One of the liver's key functions is the production of the factors (enzymes) involved in the clotting cascade. This in turn can influence the efficacy of drugs that act to influence that cascade, especially if liver function is impaired. Warfarin is an important drug to consider in this context. The use of sedative drugs in patients with hepatic impairment can increase the risk of hepatic encephalopathy and requires caution.

Drug choice

A great many drugs will undergo degrees of hepatic metabolism before elimination. Knowledge of the pharmacokinetics of a drug will therefore influence decision making if there is evidence of hepatic impairment. Selection of a drug that does not undergo (or undergoes minimal) hepatic metabolism may be more appropriate for patients with impaired liver function. For example, the antipsychotic amisulpride is not significantly metabolised by the liver and therefore does not require dosing adjustment in patients with hepatic impairment. Drugs that are more water soluble, and therefore more easily eliminated by the kidney without the need for biotransformation (metabolism), may be more appropriate.

Consideration that a drug may be hepatotoxic should also be borne in mind, especially if the patient demonstrates evidence of hepatic impairment.

Rapid Medicines Management for Healthcare Professionals, First Edition. Paul Deslandes, Simon Young and Ben Pitcher.
© 2020 John Wiley & Sons Ltd. Published 2020 by John Wiley & Sons Ltd.

Example of the impact of hepatic impairment on medication choice

Diazepam is used to manage alcohol withdrawal. Unfortunately, the metabolism of diazepam (and its active metabolites) is dependent on hepatic function. Extremes of alcohol misuse can severely compromise hepatic function. In cases of more severe hepatic compromise, the implementation of Clinical Institute Withdrawal Assessment for alcohol needs to be carefully considered because the risk of accumulation of diazepam and its active metabolites is increased.

Drug dosing

In severe liver disease pharmacological intervention should be kept to the lowest level possible. This may include the use of other (non-pharmacological) interventions where appropriate and keeping drug doses as low as possible. Inconsiderate prescribing that does not take into account the degree of hepatic impairment may result in:

1. further hepatic damage
2. accumulation of the drug in plasma and the exposure of the patient to toxic levels of the drug and increased risks of adverse effects
3. damage to other organs/tissues due to the accumulation of the parent drug and metabolites (which may also be toxic).

26 Drugs in Renal Impairment

The kidney plays a significant role in the pharmacokinetics of many drugs and changes in renal function can affect absorption, distribution, metabolism, and elimination. Patients with renal impairment may therefore be more susceptible to the adverse effects of medicines. This may necessitate dosing alterations. Physiological changes linked to renal impairment such as electrolyte disturbance may also affect the response to certain drugs (e.g. digoxin), whilst some may be ineffective in patients with renal impairment. As renal function declines with age, it is important to remember that the elderly may be particularly affected by these changes.

In addition to alterations in a medicine's effectiveness and tolerability, it should also be noted that medicines may cause toxicity to the kidney or affect kidney function. This may occur in the context of pre-existing renal impairment, requiring the medicine to be used with particular caution or avoided in such patients. However, nephrotoxic effects may also occur in patients with normal renal function, and an awareness of the likely causative drugs is necessary to identify and manage these effectively.

Assessing renal function

Renal function is typically estimated using measures such as estimated glomerular filtration rate (eGFR), or creatinine clearance. These can be derived using equations such as the modification of diet in renal disease (MDRD) and Cockroft and Gault formulae, which take into account a patient's age, sex, ethnicity, and biochemical findings. Alterations in a medicine's dosing may be made on the basis of a reduction in eGFR or creatinine clearance. However, it is important to note that these measures are only estimates of renal function and for certain medicines dosing adjustments should be made using an accurate glomerular filtration rate measurement.

Alterations in pharmacokinetics

If renal function is impaired, the elimination of many medicines from the body can be reduced. The resulting increase in plasma level can lead to adverse effects. This is particularly problematic for medicines with a narrow therapeutic range and where inactivation of the medicine through metabolic pathways does not occur (hence the drug is excreted unchanged). Dosing alterations are required for many medicines and are typically made on the basis of the degree of renal impairment. Some commonly used medicines which may require dosage adjustment in patients with renal impairment include opioids (e.g. fentanyl, morphine, etc.), oral anticoagulants, certain oral blood glucose lowering medicines (e.g. metformin, some sulphonylureas, and gliptins, e.g. saxagliptin), antibacterials (e.g. aminoglycoside antibiotics and vancomycin – note that the oral formulation of vancomycin typically has minimal bioavailability and dose reduction may not be required), digoxin, lithium, methotrexate, and other immunosuppressants,

Rapid Medicines Management for Healthcare Professionals, First Edition. Paul Deslandes, Simon Young and Ben Pitcher.
© 2020 John Wiley & Sons Ltd. Published 2020 by John Wiley & Sons Ltd.

and the antipsychotics risperidone and paliperidone. Note that this list is not exhaustive and you should refer to product information or the *British National Formulary* for further details.

If a medicine is required to be passed into the lumen of the nephron in order to exert its effect, it may no longer be effective when glomerular filtration is reduced. Such medicines should therefore be avoided, depending upon the degree of renal impairment. Examples include the antibiotic nitrofurantoin (typically used in the treatment of urinary tract infections) and the sodium glucose co-transporter 2 inhibitors (the "gliflozin" group of blood glucose lowering drugs, e.g. dapagliflozin and empagliflozin).

Medicines affecting renal function

Glomerular filtration is dependent upon blood flow through the kidney, which can be affected by a number of factors, such as cardiac output and blood volume as well as vasodilatation and vasoconstriction. Medicines that affect homeostatic mechanisms concerned with these factors may reduce glomerular filtration and have been associated with acute kidney injury. Examples include angiotensin-converting enzyme inhibitors (e.g. ramipril) and angiotensin receptor blockers (e.g. losartan), which can lead to a reduction in blood volume as well as vasodilatation of efferent renal blood vessels, diuretics, and non-steroidal anti-inflammatory drugs (NSAIDs, e.g. ibuprofen and naproxen). Use of these agents has been associated with acute kidney injury, and the risk may be increased where fluid volume is decreased or where these medicines are used in combination.

Medicines causing nephrotoxicity

In addition to reducing renal perfusion, medicines may also have a nephrotoxic effect by causing damage to other kidney tissues. One such effect is known as interstitial nephritis and may be acute or chronic in nature. Acute interstitial nephritis can result from a hypersensitivity reaction to certain medicines (as well as to infection), which leads to inflammatory processes and cellular damage in the kidney. Some examples of commonly used medicines associated with this include NSAIDs, antibiotics (including penicillins, cephalosporins, and quinolones), diuretics, and proton pump inhibitors. Chronic interstitial nephritis can occur with longer-term use of analgesics such as NSAIDs and paracetamol, lithium, and certain immunosuppressant medicines.

Medicines may also result in nephrotoxicity through other mechanisms. Examples of such nephrotoxic medicines include aminoglycoside antibiotics (e.g. gentamicin), vancomycin, the antifungal agent amphotericin, chemotherapy agents, and radiographic contrast media. These lists are not exhaustive, and further details should be obtained from the summary of product characteristics or other specialist sources. It should also be noted that any use of combinations of medicines that adversely affect renal function is likely to increase the risk of renal impairment or toxicity.

27 Biologic Medicines

What are biologic medicines?

The majority of medicines in use today are small, synthetic molecules that are made using a chemical process. Some of these are based on substances found in plants (such as the opioids pethidine and fentanyl), but it is still possible to synthesise these medicines from chemicals in a laboratory.

Biologic medicines are different. Instead of being synthesised using a chemical process, these medicines are large, complex molecules that are created in biological cells. The cells used to produce the medicine are grown in cultures and may be bacterial cells that have undergone genetic modification or modified cells of the mammalian immune system. The molecules that they produce may be copies of existing human proteins or altogether new entities.

To produce copies of existing proteins, additional DNA can be inserted into the genome of a cell line (recombinant DNA), resulting in expression of the desired protein. This process is used to produce recombinant insulin (e.g. Humulin®). Another option is to exploit the ability of the immune system to produce antibodies to foreign proteins as part of the body's defence mechanism. Immune cells are exposed to the desired target and produce an antibody that can bind to this specific target (a monoclonal antibody [Mab]). This forms the basis of many biological medicines, which can be identified from the suffix 'mab' at the end of their name.

A third type of biological medicine is known as a fusion protein. Here, two proteins are linked together (fused) so that one part of the molecule is able to bind to a specific target, whilst the other part either inactivates the target or helps to ensure that the binding site remains stable in the body. These medicines typically have the suffix 'cept'.

Some commonly used examples

Some of the earliest biological medicines to be used were recombinant insulin and erythropoietin. These were designed to mimic naturally occurring proteins found in the body. Some examples of biologic medicines, their molecular target, and their therapeutic use are shown in Table 27.1.

From the early 2000s onwards, a number of Mab medicines have been approved for human use. Mabs may combine aspects of mouse and human antibodies to form chimeric Mabs and humanised Mabs, or may be fully human. These can be identified by the suffix in the name of the medicine, and examples are shown in the table below. This is a rapidly evolving field with many new medicines being licensed with different mechanisms of action used for a variety of different indications.

Examples of fusion proteins licensed for use in the UK include abatacept, aflibercept, and etanercept.

Rapid Medicines Management for Healthcare Professionals, First Edition. Paul Deslandes, Simon Young and Ben Pitcher.
© 2020 John Wiley & Sons Ltd. Published 2020 by John Wiley & Sons Ltd.

Table 27.1 Some examples of biologic medicines, their molecular target, and their therapeutic use.

Type	Suffix	Medicine	Target	Use
Chimeric	-ximab	Abciximab	Glycoprotein iib/iiia	Inhibits platelet aggregation
		Brentuximab vedotin	CD30	Cancer
		Cetuximab	EGFR	Cancer
		Infliximab	TNFα	Arthritis/Crohn's disease
		Rituximab	CD20	Cancer/arthritis
Humanised	-zumab	Alemtuzumab	CD52	Multiple sclerosis
		Certolizumab pegol	TNFα	Arthritis/psoriasis
		Omalizumab	IgE	Asthma
		Pembrolizumab	PD-1	Cancer
		Reslizumab	IL-5	Asthma
		Tocilizumab	IL-6 receptor	Arthritis
		Trastuzumab	EGFR (HER2)	Cancer
Human	-umab	Adalimumab	TNFα	Arthritis/psoriasis/IBD/uveitis
		Evolocumab	PCSK9	Hypercholesterolaemia
		Golimumab	TNFα	Arthritis/IBD
		Ipilimumab	CTLA-4	Cancer
		Nivolumab	PD-1	Cancer
		Secukinumab	Interleukin-17A	Arthritis/psoriasis
		Ustekinumab	Interleukin-12/23	IBD

EGFR, epidermal growth factor receptor; TNFα, tumour necrosis factor-alpha; IgE, immunoglobulin E; IL, interleukin; IBD, inflammatory bowel disease.

How do they work?

Biologic medicines such as recombinant insulin and erythropoietin act by mimicking the body's own endogenous versions of these molecules. Mabs and fusion proteins act on a range of signalling molecules and receptors in the body. However, the aim of these medicines is to be selective in the molecules that they target, unlike a traditional small molecule medicine (e.g. amitriptyline), which might bind to a number of different targets, resulting in side effects.

Mabs targeting signalling molecules (e.g. interleukins and tumour necrosis factor) typically interfere with the binding of the molecule to its receptor, thereby preventing it from eliciting its usual response. Mabs targeting receptors (e.g. PD-1) bind to the receptor and prevent the action of the endogenous signalling molecule. This is similar to the action of a more traditional receptor antagonist.

The fusion proteins available in the UK bind to an endogenous signalling molecule, preventing it from binding to its receptor and eliciting a response. This is similar to the action of certain Mabs. Examples include abatacept (which binds to CD80 and CD86), aflibercept (which binds to vascular endothelial growth factor A and placental growth factor), and etanercept (which binds to tumour necrosis factor-alpha [TNFα]).

What conditions are they used to treat?

Biologic medicines are licensed to treat a range of conditions from cancer to hypercholesterolaemia. Medicines targeting inflammatory mediators such as TNFα and interleukins are typically used in the treatment of arthritis and inflammatory bowel disease. Immune system modulators such as nivolumab and pembrolizumab are used in the treatment of cancers. The same medicine may be licensed for multiple indications (e.g. adalimumab).

How are they given?

Because these are large molecules, these medicines cannot typically be given orally. Exposure to digestive enzymes in the stomach would result in degradation of the drug, whilst the size of the molecule would prohibit absorption through the gastrointestinal mucosa. As a result, parenteral administration either by intravenous infusion or subcutaneous injection is typically used. Oral preparations for the treatment of inflammatory bowel disease that deliver the medicine to the intestinal mucosa are in development. The Mabs and fusion proteins are long acting and can typically be given on a weekly or sometimes less frequent basis.

What are the adverse effects?

Anaphylactic reactions can occur during the administration of biologic medicines, particularly in patients with a previous history of certain allergies. As many of these medicines target aspects of the immune system, there is an increased risk of serious infections and a risk of transplant rejection with certain biologics. For further information on adverse effects consult the product literature.

What are biosimilar medicines?

When the patent for a medicine expires, it is possible for a company other than the company that developed the medicine to produce a copy. For traditional small molecule medicines these are known as a 'generic' versions. Because they are produced by chemical synthesis, an exact copy of the original medicine can be made relatively easily. However, this is not the case with biologic medicines. Due to the complexity of the manufacturing process and of the drug molecule itself, it is not possible to produce an exact copy of the original medicine. Instead, a molecule with a similar molecular structure and similar pharmacological properties can be produced, and this is termed a biosimilar medicine.

Advanced therapies

As discussed above, traditional biologic medicines are produced from cultured cells. However, it is also possible to utilise a patient's own cells to produce a medicine. This process involves harvesting some of the desired cells (these may be stem cells or tissue cells) from a patient, growing them in a laboratory to increase their number, and reimplanting them into the patient. In the UK, the National Institute for Health and Care Excellence has recommended that a number of such therapies should be available for use. These include autologous chondrocyte implantation involving cartilage cells to treat knee damage and autologous corneal cells to treat eye burns. It is also possible to genetically modify the cells removed from the patient prior to reimplantation in order to 'reprogram' them for a specific purpose. This forms the basis of Strimvelis®, used to treat adenosine deaminase deficiency, and chimeric antigen receptor therapies (CAR-T) such as Kymriah®, which utilise modified T-cells to treat cancer. CAR-T treatments may offer a cure for certain cancers, although the cost is currently high and raises questions of affordability for healthcare funders.

28 Pharmacogenetics

What are pharmacogenetics and pharmacogenomics?

Pharmacogenetics and pharmacogenomics are areas of science that examine the way in which a person's genetic characteristics affect their response to medicines. Pharmacogenetics looks at the impact of a specific gene whereas pharmacogenomics looks at the entire genetic profile of an individual. As our understanding of the way in which genetic variation influences treatment outcome increases, it is likely that the medicines that we use will become more and more tailored to individual patients.

How can pharmacogenomics be applied to current treatment?

Current applications of pharmacogenomics include the ability to predict which patients are likely to respond to certain treatments, which patients are likely to experience adverse effects, and how patients metabolise certain drugs.

Treatment response

The response of some patients to the effects of the anticoagulant warfarin may be determined by genetic variation. Warfarin inhibits an enzyme known as vitamin K epoxide reductase. Different patients may have slightly different forms of this enzyme, and the form that they have is determined by a gene called vitamin K epoxide reductase component 1 (VKOR1). Patients with one form may respond to a different dose of warfarin than those with another form.

Examples of the practical application of pharmacogenomics include determining whether patients with cancer are likely to respond to treatment. The response to certain medicines in the treatment of melanoma and non-small cell lung cancer may be dependent upon the presence of a mutation in the BRAF gene. The medicine dabrafenib is indicated for the treatment of these cancers when the BRAF V600 mutation is present. Identification of this mutation is required before treatment with dabrafenib can be initiated. Similarly, the presence of epidermal growth factor receptor mutation determines whether patients with non-small cell lung cancer are eligible for treatment with osimertinib.

Adverse effects

The incidence of certain adverse effects to medicines may also be genetically determined. Variation in alleles of the human leukocyte antigen-B (HLA-B) gene can help to predict the occurrence of severe skin rashes to certain medicines, in particular the anticonvulsant

Rapid Medicines Management for Healthcare Professionals, First Edition. Paul Deslandes, Simon Young and Ben Pitcher.
© 2020 John Wiley & Sons Ltd. Published 2020 by John Wiley & Sons Ltd.

carbamazepine. Similarly, phenytoin sensitivity may be predicted by variation in HLA-B as well as the compliment factor H related 4 gene (CFHR4). It is also believed that the incidence of cough associated with angiotensin converting enzyme inhibitors may be a product of gene polymorphism.

Drug metabolism

A number of drugs undergo metabolism through the cytochrome P450 (CYP450) enzyme system in the liver. There are a number of different CYP450 enzyme families, and the activity of some of these, including the 2D6 type, is linked to genetic polymorphism. As a result, the population can be divided into those who are 'poor' metabolisers through this enzyme, those who are 'intermediate' metabolisers, those who are 'extensive' metabolisers, and those who are 'ultra-rapid' metabolisers.

This variation can lead to increased or decreased plasma levels of a given drug in different individuals (even if the same dose is administered). CYP2D6 plays an important role in the metabolism of some antidepressants and antipsychotics. Poor metabolisers would be expected to have a reduced ability to metabolise the drug and therefore experience higher plasma levels with the potential for adverse effects. Ultra-rapid metabolisers would be expected to have an increased ability to metabolise the drug and therefore experience lower plasma levels with the potential for treatment failure. However, there are also circumstances where the reverse is true. Ultra-rapid metabolism has been associated with toxicity related to the opioid codeine. This is because codeine is metabolised to the more potent opioid morphine by CYP2D6 enzymes. Individuals who are ultra-rapid metabolisers are more effective at converting codeine to morphine, leading to increased morphine levels and associated toxicity. Conversely, poor metabolisers are less able to convert codeine to morphine and may not derive significant benefit from codeine use.

29 Adverse Drug Reactions

What is an adverse drug reaction?

An adverse drug reaction (ADR) was defined by Edwards and Aronson (*Lancet*, 2000; 356:1255–59) as 'an appreciably harmful or unpleasant reaction, resulting from an intervention related to the use of a medicinal product, which predicts hazard from future administration and warrants prevention or specific treatment, or alteration of the dosage regimen, or withdrawal of the product.'

This definition encompasses adverse effects of medicines that may be related to the active drug component, or to one or more of the excipients used in the medicine formulation (e.g. nut oils used in the formulation of certain long-acting antipsychotic injections).

What are the different types of ADR?

ADRs have typically been classified into type A or type B depending upon the properties of the drug. An extended classification system (including types C–F) has also been used to define ADRs that cannot be readily classified into these two groups.

Type A ADRs are typically described as **A**ugmented (increased) effects of a drug when used within the therapeutic dose range, and which are related to the drug's pharmacological effects. As a result, these ADRs tend to be common and predictable, with a low chance of mortality. Type A ADRs may result from the drug's pharmacological effect being exerted through its intended mechanism of action, e.g. salbutamol may be associated with tachycardia due to agonism at beta-receptors. However, they may also result from an effect through a mechanism of action unrelated to the therapeutic effect, e.g. constipation seen with certain antipsychotics. Type A ADRs may be more common in patients with altered pharmacokinetics (e.g. the elderly) and with medicines with a narrow therapeutic range (e.g. lithium).

Type B reactions were traditionally considered **B**izarre and unrelated to a drug's known pharmacological effects. However, as our understanding of the underpinning physiology and pharmacology has increased, these reactions have become better defined and characterised. Such effects are typically mediated through immunological processes, are rare and unpredictable, and can be life threatening. Examples and some of the causative agents include the following:

- Anaphylaxis presents with symptoms such as angioedema and bronchoconstriction (typically associated with penicillins, other antibiotics, and biologic monoclonal antibodies).
- Severe skin reactions (e.g. Stevens–Johnson syndrome and toxic epidermal necrolysis) present with ulceration or severe skin rash with loss of skin, respectively (typically associated with anticonvulsants, but may occur with other drugs including [but not limited to] non-steroidal anti-inflammatory drugs [NSAIDs] and some antibiotics).

Rapid Medicines Management for Healthcare Professionals, First Edition. Paul Deslandes, Simon Young and Ben Pitcher.
© 2020 John Wiley & Sons Ltd. Published 2020 by John Wiley & Sons Ltd.

- ADRs affecting the liver and kidney may be mediated through immunological processes (associated with certain antibiotics, allopurinol, and NSAIDs as well as other drugs).
- Drug rash with eosinophilia and systemic symptoms (DRESS) syndrome may affect several organ systems (including skin and liver), and has been associated with certain anticonvulsants, allopurinol, and other drugs.

ADRs type C–F include those reactions that result from Chronic use of a medicine, occur after a Delayed period of time, occur at the End of treatment, or involve treatment Failure. Type C (chronic) effects occur with cumulative use of a medicine over a prolonged period of time (e.g. osteonecrosis of the jaw following treatment with bisphosphonates). Type D (delayed) ADRs occur some time after exposure to the medicine. Type E reactions are withdrawal effects that occur at the end of treatment with the associated medicine (e.g. following opioid or benzodiazepine withdrawal). Type F refers to treatment failure, which may be associated with drug interactions, for example when a cytochrome P450 enzyme inducer is taken in combination with another medicine.

An alternate system of ADR classification is the DoTS system. This was designed to characterise the reaction and capture factors influencing it, rather than focusing on the properties of the medicine. The key aspects are the dose at which the reaction occurs (Do), the timing of its appearance (T), and patient characteristics affecting susceptibility (S). The reaction can then be described in relation to these three factors.

The ADR may be seen at subtherapeutic doses (i.e. hypersensitivity), at therapeutic doses, or at supratherapeutic (toxic) doses. It may be time dependent, occurring early in treatment or with repeated exposure to the medicine. Alternatively, the ADR may be unrelated to the treatment duration (time independent), occurring due to a change in dose or a change in pharmacokinetic or pharmacodynamic factors. Increased susceptibility may be related to age (e.g. declining renal function in the elderly), sex, genetic variation (e.g. presence of HLA-B*15:02 allele in South-East Asian populations leading to increased risk of Stevens–Johnson syndrome with carbamazepine), ethnicity and co-morbidity.

How are ADRs identified?

There are a number of different approaches to identify ADRs. The more common Type A reactions can be detected during the early clinical trials of a medicine that take place during the development process. However, due to the relatively small number of people who receive a medicine during early clinical trials and their typically short-term nature, less common reactions and those requiring prolonged exposure to treatment are unlikely to be identified. Post-marketing trials of a medicine involving larger patient populations are more likely to reveal less common ADRs, whilst observational studies (e.g. case control and cohort studies – see Chapter 82 for further information) may help to identify associations between medicines and certain ADRs.

Following the thalidomide disaster in the mid twentieth century, the importance of a co-ordinated mechanism to learn from spontaneously reported ADRs was recognised. In the UK, the Yellow Card reporting scheme was established to facilitate reporting of suspected ADRs by healthcare professionals and patients. This scheme allows suspected ADRs to be reported to a central body (the Medicines and Healthcare Products Regulatory Agency), who liaise with other similar organisations to detect trends that can suggest a potential problem with a given medicine. The effectiveness of this system relies upon the level of reporting. Under-reporting of suspected ADRs remains a limitation despite campaigns and changes to the process to facilitate greater reporting. All healthcare professionals as well as patients, relatives, and carers are therefore encouraged to report any suspected ADR, particularly those that are serious in nature, those associated with new medicines or those under increased scrutiny as indicated by the black triangle symbol (▼) on product information.

How can ADRs be managed?

Type A ADRs usually resolve following dose reduction or discontinuation of the causal medicine. Where this is not possible, a second medicine may sometimes be prescribed to treat the ADR, although this can lead to inappropriate polypharmacy.

Immune-mediated (type B) ADRs may be more severe and may require inpatient admission. Treatment will include discontinuation of the causative agent and possible administration of medicines to reduce any allergic response or provide symptomatic relief. Such medicines may include corticosteroids or antihistamines to attenuate allergic response, or adrenaline/epinephrine for anaphylaxis.

Where a patient has been identified as experiencing a serious ADR in response to a particular medicine, prevention of future exposure is important. This requires accurate documentation of the causative medicine and the nature of the ADR, and the transfer of this information between care settings when required. It should be noted that many patients who describe allergic reactions to medicines such as penicillin may not have a true anaphylactic response to exposure. This may result in inappropriate prescribing of alternative agents in the future, and highlights the need for accurate and detailed documentation.

30 Drug Interactions

What is a drug–drug interaction?

A drug interaction can be defined as an effect exerted by one medicine on another medicine when the two are taken together.

Do interactions only involve medicines?

No, the effects of certain medicines may be influenced by foods and other substances administered to the body.

What types of drug interaction are there?

Drug interactions can broadly be divided into pharmacodynamic and pharmacokinetic interactions, depending upon the underlying pharmacological mechanism. However, it is possible to see both types of interaction when two medicines are combined.

What are pharmacodynamic drug interactions?

A pharmacodynamic interaction occurs when a patient is taking two (or more) medicines that mediate additive or opposing physiological effects. This may occur as a result of competition for the same site of action (such as a receptor), or through different pharmacological mechanisms. The result of the interaction may be to enhance the effect of the medicines or to reduce the effect of the medicines.

Administering two medicines (or a medicine and another substance) that results in an increased effect at a given site of action will augment their effects. This may help to enhance the therapeutic effect, for example combining carbidopa with amantadine, both of which affect dopamine neurotransmission for the treatment of Parkinson's disease. It may also lead to an increased risk of adverse drug reactions, such as combining alcohol with benzodiazepines leading to increased sedation. Another important example of a medicine combination resulting in an additive risk of adverse effects through similar pharmacodynamic properties is prolongation of the cardiac QT interval. This may result in potentially fatal arrhythmias and has been associated with certain antipsychotics, erythromycin, methadone, and many other medicines, particularly when they are used in combination.

Medicines may also produce an increased physiological effect by acting through different parts of a common process. For example, platelet activation leading to blood clotting involves a number of different chemical mediators. Non-steroidal anti-inflammatory drugs (NSAIDs), selective serotonin re-uptake inhibitors, and warfarin all reduce clotting through different mechanisms and when used together increase the risk of bleeding.

Rapid Medicines Management for Healthcare Professionals, First Edition. Paul Deslandes, Simon Young and Ben Pitcher.
© 2020 John Wiley & Sons Ltd. Published 2020 by John Wiley & Sons Ltd.

Administering a medicine that is an antagonist at a given receptor with a medicine that is an agonist at the same receptor may lead to a reduced effect. For example, naloxone (an opioid receptor antagonist) reduces the effects of morphine (an opioid receptor agonist) and is therefore used to treat opioid overdose. However, as with additive effects, opposing effects may be mediated through different pharmacodynamic mechanisms. For example, NSAIDs cause an increase in blood pressure due to increased fluid retention and may therefore oppose the actions of antihypertensive agents such as vasodilator calcium channel blockers.

What are pharmacokinetic interactions?

A pharmacokinetic interaction occurs when one medicine (or other substance) affects the pharmacokinetics of another medicine. The result of the interaction will be to increase or decrease the plasma level of one (or both) of the medicines, which may lead to a change in the therapeutic or adverse effects. An interaction resulting in increased plasma levels may lead to an increased risk of adverse drug reactions or toxicity, whilst an interaction resulting in reduced plasma levels may lead to a loss of therapeutic effect. Interactions may occur at any of the stages of absorption, distribution, metabolism or elimination, although the clinical significance of each may vary.

Pharmacokinetic interactions involving absorption

Pharmacokinetic interactions involving absorption are generally associated with oral administration and may lead to an increase or decrease in bioavailability. These interactions may result from a chemical reaction between two medicines making one less soluble and less well absorbed, changes in the pH or motility of the gastrointestinal tract, or changes in the effects of metabolic enzymes in the wall of the gastrointestinal tract (see the section on pharmacokinetic interactions involving metabolism). Chemical reactions can occur between antacids containing metal ions (e.g. aluminium, calcium, magnesium) and certain antibiotics (e.g. tetracycline), leading to reduced bioavailability of the antibiotic. Metal ions are also found in milk, therefore a similar interaction can also be seen between milk and tetracycline. Medicines that increase the pH of the stomach can affect the absorption of some medicines (e.g. ketoconazole) by reducing their solubility, whilst medicines altering gastrointestinal motility (e.g. muscarinic receptor blockers) may increase or decrease the absorption of other medicines.

Pharmacokinetic interactions involving distribution

Pharmacokinetic interactions involving distribution often involve the displacement of a drug from a plasma protein binding site. Whilst this effect can lead to increased plasma levels, the effect is usually short lived due to increased metabolism and elimination of the affected drug. As a result, there is usually little change in clinical effect. Other interactions involving distribution include alterations in brain penetration of certain medicines due to inhibition of transport proteins. Medicines inhibiting the effect of p-glycoprotein transporters can increase levels of loperamide in the brain with the potential to result in effects on the central nervous system, which are not typically seen with this medicine.

Pharmacokinetic interactions involving metabolism

Many medicines undergo metabolism in the liver, mediated by enzymes including the cytochrome P450 (CYP450) family. The activity of certain CYP450 enzymes can be influenced by medicines, foods, and other substances, which may increase or decrease their activity. Increasing the activity of the enzymes can reduce the plasma levels of the medicines that they metabolise, whilst decreasing the activity of the enzymes can increase the plasma levels of the medicines that they metabolise. CYP450 enzymes are also found in the wall of the gastrointestinal tract and, similarly, increasing or decreasing their activity can decrease or increase a medicine's bioavailability accordingly. Examples of medicines and other substances that increase CYP450 activity include carbamazepine, phenytoin, rifampicin, and hydrocarbons in tobacco smoke, all of which can reduce the plasma levels of certain medicines. This may result in therapeutic failure. Examples of medicines that inhibit (decrease) CYP450 activity include some macrolide antibacterials (e.g. erythromycin, clarithromycin), some antifungals (e.g. fluconazole, ketoconazole), and some antidepressants (e.g. fluoxetine, paroxetine). These medicines may therefore increase the plasma levels of other medicines, which may result in increased adverse effects or toxicity. Other substances that inhibit CYP450 activity include grapefruit juice, which can increase the bioavailability of certain calcium channel blockers, and certain statins, which may necessitate dosage alteration.

Pharmacokinetic interactions involving elimination

Pharmacokinetic interactions involving elimination may result from drug-induced changes in renal (kidney) function. Many medicines are eliminated via the kidney, and alterations in renal blood flow and the activity of renal transport proteins can result in interactions. NSAIDs can reduce renal perfusion and inhibit transport proteins, resulting in increased plasma concentrations of lithium and methotrexate. As both lithium and methotrexate have narrow therapeutic ranges, this interaction may result in toxicity.

Clinical implications of drug interactions

The *British National Formulary* (BNF) gives an indication of whether an interaction has been observed in practice, or whether it is based upon a theoretical extrapolation of the drug's characteristics. This may help to guide prescribers and other healthcare professionals in safe and effective medicines management decision making. From a clinical perspective, the BNF also considers interactions on the basis of their potential severity with respect to patient outcome (severe, moderate, or mild). Those classified as severe may be life-threatening or result in permanent detrimental effects, whilst those which are mild are unlikely to cause serious concern.

Decisions regarding the appropriateness of treating patients with medicines that interact should be made on a case-by-case basis, evaluating the potential risks and benefits.

31 Drug Allergy and Anaphylaxis

Allergy to a drug is a form of adverse drug reaction, specifically a type B or 'bizarre' reaction. A drug allergy is an immune response mediated through histamine and other chemicals, where the body identifies the drug as an antigen and over-reacts to it.

Types of reaction

Drug allergies can manifest in lots of different ways. Some of the most common include a skin rash (urticaria) or mucosal changes. The reaction can be limited to the localised area around the site of exposure or may manifest systemically across the body. Reactions may manifest relatively quickly (within an hour of exposure) or have a delayed onset (days to weeks later). The reaction may not occur on the first exposure to the drug but following subsequent doses.

In some individuals, the reaction may escalate and include a systemic response such as vasodilation or reactions away from the site of exposure, such as bronchospasm (particularly in patients with asthma). These systemic reactions can progress into the serious condition known as anaphylaxis. In this situation, the vasodilation and swelling associated with an inflammatory response results in a redistribution of body fluids out of the circulatory system and into the extracellular fluid, which can result in excessive widespread swelling that can be particularly dangerous around the neck and face (angioedema), making breathing difficult or even impossible. The loss of fluid from the circulating volume can also produce dangerous loss of blood pressure. Anaphylactic shock is a dangerous, life-threatening situation that must be addressed urgently.

Parenteral medications, such as creams or injections, may produce more localised reaction at the site of administration, but if a patient is very allergic to the drug it could still progress into a full systemic reaction.

Incidence

Drug allergies are not especially common but due to the large number of drugs administered to patients and the significant potential for harm, they should be an important consideration and always checked before any drug is prescribed or administered.

Some commonly used drugs have a surprisingly high incidence of allergy. Non-steroidal anti-inflammatory drug allergy has been reported as occurring in up to 10% of the population. Penicillin-based antibiotics are famous for their potential to cause allergic reactions. However, whilst approximately 10% of the population report that they are allergic to penicillin, it is believed that only 1–2% actually have a true allergy. Many misidentify themselves as having an allergy due to experiencing another form of adverse reaction (such as nausea or diarrhoea). This is unfortunate as they may well be precluding themselves from receiving

Rapid Medicines Management for Healthcare Professionals, First Edition. Paul Deslandes, Simon Young and Ben Pitcher.
© 2020 John Wiley & Sons Ltd. Published 2020 by John Wiley & Sons Ltd.

optimal treatment in the future and this may result in the use of more expensive or less effective alternatives.

Management of allergy

If a patient appears to be manifesting an allergic reaction it needs to be managed promptly. The exact details of how to manage serious allergic reactions such as anaphylaxis are outlined in detail by the Resuscitation Council (www.resus.org.uk) and centre around the administration of adrenaline, oxygen, and i/v fluids as soon as possible.

Outlined below is a discussion of some of the interventions and strategies used to prevent and treat allergies and anaphylaxis.

Avoidance of allergen

The most effective way of managing drug allergy is to ensure that the patient is not exposed to that drug. If a patient is allergic to a drug it should be recorded in the patient's notes and usually on their drug chart. However, documentation can be poor and the transfer of information between care settings unreliable. Guidelines for the documentation of suspected allergic reactions can be found in NICE clinical guideline CG183, available at www.nice.org.uk/guidance/cg183/resources/drug-allergy-diagnosis-and-management-pdf-35109811022821.

In secondary care facilities (e.g. hospitals), patients may be given a band to wear on their wrist to identify that they are allergic to a drug. However, the absence of a band should not be taken as a guarantee that they have no allergy. This should be verbally checked with the patient (if possible) before any drug is prescribed or administered. If a patient appears to be presenting with an allergic response to a drug being administered, this should be discontinued immediately.

Antihistamines (e.g. chlorphenamine, cetirizine)

Allergy is a histamine-mediated response, which means the various manifestations of the allergy (vasodilation, swelling, itching, etc.) are produced by histamine acting upon its receptors (H_1 receptors) in the various tissues of the body. If the histamine H_1 receptor is blocked by an antagonist, it can lessen or even prevent the allergic reaction. Antihistamines (such as oral cetirizine) may be effective in localised allergy. However, whilst antihistamines (typically intravenous chlorphenamine) are used in anaphylaxis, they will not be sufficient to completely control the reaction and will not be the first-line option.

Adrenaline

Adrenaline is naturally produced as part of the sympathetic nervous system. It is the first-line treatment for serious anaphylactic reactions of any type (most widely known for its use in adrenaline auto-injectors to relieve anaphylaxis due to food allergy). The action of adrenaline is mostly attributed to its established effects of bronchodilation and vasoconstriction, reducing the displacement of fluid into the tissues and restoring blood pressure.

Steroids (e.g. hydrocortisone)

Steroids are powerful anti-inflammatory drugs and are included in the treatment regime for anaphylactic reactions. They appear to be useful in reducing or preventing continuing (biphasic) reactions.

Therapeutics

32 Therapeutics Chapter Template

Section 3 of this book explores some of the drugs and drug groups commonly used in clinical practice. Each of the chapters follows a similar layout, which is described in this chapter. It was not possible to include all of the available drugs or drug groups in this section, therefore we have also included a blank template for you to fill in yourself for a drug or drug group that is relevant to your practice.

Commonly used examples
Each chapter will include examples of some of the more common drugs from this group. This will not be an exhaustive list.

Are these drugs all the same?
Whilst the drugs in each chapter will follow a certain theme, there will be differences between the different drugs being discussed. This section will therefore discuss if there are any fundamental differences which result in the drugs being grouped or used in different ways.

What are these drugs used to treat?
A simple explanation of what condition(s) the drug in question might be used to treat.

What do these drugs do?
An outline of how the drug in question treats the condition it is indicated for.

What's the difference between different types?
Different drugs will have different properties (good and bad). This section will explore these differences to help understand why one drug may be chosen over another.

How are these drugs given?
Any particular points to consider regarding the possible routes of administration.

Rapid Medicines Management for Healthcare Professionals, First Edition. Paul Deslandes, Simon Young and Ben Pitcher.
© 2020 John Wiley & Sons Ltd. Published 2020 by John Wiley & Sons Ltd.

Dosing

Whilst specific doses should be obtained from clinical sources such as the *British National Formulary* (BNF), this section will discuss any specific issues related to how the drug is dosed, for example if it is dosed by weight or age.

What are the notable adverse effects to look out for?

Almost all drugs have adverse effects and a comprehensive list can be found in the BNF or in the summary of product characteristics (SmPC) for the drug in question. The intention of this section is to raise awareness of particular or problematic side effects.

Hypersensitivity and anaphylaxis are technically possible adverse effects of any drug, but this will only be discussed if it is particularly notable (e.g. penicillin-based antibiotics).

How can the adverse effects be minimised?

This section will explore any strategies that may be employed to avoid or reduce problematic adverse effects. These might include timing of doses or the use of other medicines to alleviate symptoms of adverse effects.

What needs to be monitored?

This section is a discussion of things that may need to be monitored or assessed before or during the use of a drug. This may include some form of specific assay, such as serum potassium or international normalised ratio, or it could involve monitoring a patient's vital signs, such as blood pressure or respiratory rate.

What drug interactions are important?

Some drugs have particularly notable interactions that are either very common or potentially very harmful. This section does not necessarily include an exhaustive list, but a full list of drug interactions can be found in the interactions appendix of the BNF.

Discontinuing treatment

Some drugs should not be abruptly stopped. If a drug is known to cause withdrawal effects or if there are any specific strategies regarding reducing the dose of a drug before discontinuation, they will be discussed here. However, the return of symptoms or worsening of an ongoing condition that would result from stopping treatment will not be discussed, as this can apply to many drugs.

Other considerations

Some drugs or drug groups have eccentricities that are worthy of note to ensure safe and effective use, but do not fit in the other sections.

33 Anti-emetics

Commonly used examples
Antihistamines, e.g. cinnarizine and cyclizine.
Cannabinoids, e.g. nabilone.
Dopamine receptor antagonists, e.g. domperidone, metoclopramide.
Neurokinin receptor antagonists, e.g. aprepitant.
$5HT_3$ receptor antagonists, e.g. granisetron and ondansetron.
Phenothiazines, e.g. levomepromazine, prochlorperazine.

Are these drugs all the same?
The medications/groups listed do not have one common mechanism of action: metoclopramide and domperidone block dopamine receptors (which are involved with central and peripheral triggers of nausea) and nabilone is a synthetic cannabinoid.

What are these drugs used to treat?
The medications classified as being used to treat nausea and vomiting are used for a range of indications. These include nausea and vomiting, nausea and vomiting associated with chemotherapy, in pain management/palliative care to treat nausea (this is typically nausea associated with large doses of opioids), labyrinth disorders, postoperative nausea, motion sickness, and other balance disorders.

What do these drugs do?
The exact mechanism by which antihistamines work is unclear. They have effects centrally and on lower oesophageal sphincter tone. Nabilone is a cannabinoid and the cannabinoids are believed to influence the body's emetic mechanisms. Domperidone and metoclopramide have gastrokinetic peripheral effects and an influence on the chemoreceptor trigger zone (CTZ). In addition, metoclopramide has central effects on the triggers of nausea and vomiting. Aprepitant antagonises the pharmacological effects of substance P. The vomiting centre of the brain (area postrema) contains high concentrations of substance P and antagonising its effects reduces nausea and vomiting. $5HT_3$ receptor antagonists such as ondansetron may have an effect on the release of serotonin in the small intestine (which triggers nausea) and are used for treating nausea associated with radiotherapy and chemotherapy. Phenothiazines (a family of drugs that are used in other clinical areas, such as psychiatry) such as prochlorperazine influence the activity of the CTZ and reduce nausea by blocking dopamine receptors.

Rapid Medicines Management for Healthcare Professionals, First Edition. Paul Deslandes, Simon Young and Ben Pitcher.
© 2020 John Wiley & Sons Ltd. Published 2020 by John Wiley & Sons Ltd.

How are these drugs given?

Antihistamines can be given by the oral route and also by the injectable route. Cyclizine is often delivered in syringe drivers in combination with opioids. Nabilone is available as a capsule (it is a controlled drug). Domperidone is available as tablet and oral suspension. Metoclopramide is available as an oral solution, tablet, and solution for injection. Aprepitant is available as a capsule. The $5HT_3$ antagonists are available as a variety of oral dosage forms as well as injectable, rectal, and transdermal dosage forms. Phenothiazines are typically delivered via the mouth.

Many antiemetics are available as buccal or orodispersible formulations because of the difficulty patients may have in absorbing oral formulations.

Dosing

The antiemetics are usually dosed in fixed daily doses to stem the effects of ongoing nausea and vomiting or given in doses titrated against nausea and vomiting. Many patients will take medication for nausea and vomiting after chemotherapy in a pattern that they will tailor themselves to stave off their sickness. Patients may be offered one or more of these medications depending on the nature of the nausea and vomiting.

What are the notable adverse effects to look out for?

Antihistamines can cause drowsiness and can affect the patient's ability to drive or operate heavy machinery. Cyclizine is also liable to misuse because of its euphoric and psychoactive pharmacological effects. Some antihistamines also have antimuscarinic effects and can cause dry mouth and blurred vision.

Nabilone can cause drowsiness and dizziness, euphoria, and dry mouth. It is a cannabinoid and is a substance that could be liable to misuse.

Domperidone can cause dry mouth. This medication is known to prolong the cardiac QT interval and is contraindicated in a range of hepatic, renal, and cardiac disorders. Metoclopramide can cause diarrhoea, asthenia, and drowsiness. It is known to cause extrapyramidal side effects (EPS), particularly in children, younger adults, and the elderly. There are specific limitations on the use of metoclopramide in clinical practice.

Aprepitant can cause decreased appetite, headache, constipation, dyspepsia, and fatigue.

Ondansetron can be associated with headache, a sensation of warmth/flushing, and local reactions can occur in response to injectable preparations.

The phenothiazines cause drowsiness and some antimuscarinic side effects such as dry mouth and blurred vision and may be associated with a risk of EPS.

What needs to be monitored?

This will depend upon the specific medicine, but commonly include medication adverse effects and their influence on risks such as falls, the appearance of EPS with the use of metoclopramide, and the potential misuse of medications containing cyclizine and nabilone.

What drug interactions are important?

The interactions of the medications used in nausea and vomiting are many and varied. Domperidone has many interactions because of the way it is metabolised by the liver. Drugs inhibiting certain cytochrome P450 enzymes such as erythromycin can increase domperidone levels in the body. The Medicines and Healthcare Products Regulatory Agency issued a warning concerning the use of domperidone in combination with medicines known to prolong the cardiac QT interval in 2014.

The drowsiness caused by many of the medications can be augmented by other medication or substances that can cause drowsiness, such as alcohol.

Other considerations

The use of medication for nausea and vomiting is very dependent on the cause and nature of the nausea and vomiting. Vomiting during pregnancy, vomiting caused by chemotherapy, and vomiting of unknown origin all need to be tackled in a considered way when intervening pharmacologically. One medication does not suit all conditions.

34 Antacids and Anti-Secretory Medicines

Commonly used examples

Alginates and antacids. Sodium alginate, aluminium hydroxide, magnesium hydroxide, magnesium trisilicate, potassium bicarbonate, Gaviscon®.

Histamine H_2 receptor antagonists (H₂RAs). Cimetidine, famotidine, nizatidine, ranitidine.

Proton pump inhibitors (PPIs). Esomeprazole, lansoprazole, omeprazole, pantoprazole, rabeprazole.

Are these drugs all the same?

Antacids and antisecretory medicines are divided into different groups according to their mechanism of action. Drugs from the same group have similar pharmacodynamic properties and effectiveness, but drugs from different groups vary significantly.

What are these drugs used to treat?

Antacids and antisecretory medicines reduce the acidity (increase the pH) of the stomach. The different groups of medicines are used to treat different conditions. These include a range of gastrointestinal (GI) disorders, from dyspepsia (indigestion) to more severe peptic ulcer disease and Barrett's oesophagus. They are also used to prevent peptic ulceration associated with non-steroidal anti-inflammatory drugs (NSAIDs) or stress. PPIs may be used in combination with antibacterial medicines for the eradication of *Helicobacter pylori* infection.

What do these drugs do?

Antacids increase the pH of the stomach through a simple chemical reaction. The antacid is alkaline in nature and neutralises the acidity of the stomach contents. Alginates form rafts above the stomach contents, preventing them from entering the oesophagus and causing symptoms of acid reflux.

H₂RAs and PPIs both reduce secretion of acid from parietal cells of the gastric mucosa, but this effect is achieved in different ways. H₂RAs inhibit the effect of histamine at H_2 receptors found on parietal cells. The action of histamine stimulating these receptors facilitates gastric acid release; by blocking this effect H₂RAs inhibit this process. PPIs act directly on the H^+-K^+-ATPase transporter system (the proton pump), which is responsible for the transfer of H^+ ions (acid) from the parietal cell into the gastric lumen.

Rapid Medicines Management for Healthcare Professionals, First Edition. Paul Deslandes, Simon Young and Ben Pitcher.
© 2020 John Wiley & Sons Ltd. Published 2020 by John Wiley & Sons Ltd.

How are these drugs given?

Alginates and antacids. Regularly or as required (up to three times a day and at night), by mouth for relief of symptoms of dyspepsia. Alginates should normally be taken after food.

H₂RAs. Regularly (usually twice daily), by mouth, on a short-term basis (4–8 weeks) to treat gastro-oesophageal reflux disease (GORD) or peptic ulceration.

PPIs. Regularly (usually daily), by mouth, on a short-term basis (4–8 weeks) to treat GORD or peptic ulceration. Regularly (usually twice daily), by mouth, on a short-term basis (2 weeks) in combination with antibacterials for eradication of *Helicobacter pylori*. PPIs may be given on a longer-term basis in Zollinger–Ellison syndrome, Barrett's oesophagus or to prevent NSAID-induced peptic ulceration.

Dosing

Antacids contain electrolytes, including aluminium and magnesium. In patients with renal impairment accumulation of these can lead to toxicity therefore doses should be reduced or these medicines avoided altogether.

Alginates usually contain sodium as well as calcium, magnesium or potassium. Caution is needed in patients with congestive cardiac failure, renal impairment, those on a sodium-restricted diet, and any patients in whom electrolyte disturbance would be problematic.

H₂RAs. Doses should normally be reduced in patients with renal impairment.

PPIs. Dosage adjustment may be required in hepatic or renal impairment – consult specific product literature.

What are the notable adverse effects to look out for?

This group of medicines is generally well tolerated. Alteration in gastrointestinal motility may occur. Magnesium-containing antacids as well as PPIs are commonly associated with diarrhoea, whilst aluminium-containing antacids tend to cause constipation.

Other considerations concerning their use include:

Prolonged use of any antacid may mask signs of gastric cancer and ongoing symptoms with alarm features (such as swallowing difficulties, bleeding, anaemia, weight loss) should be investigated.

PPIs. Observational studies have raised concerns over possible associations with hypo-magnesaemia, *Clostridium difficile* infection, osteoporosis, and very rarely subacute cutaneous lupus erythematosus, particularly with prolonged use.

How can the adverse effects be minimised?

All antacids should be prescribed at the lowest possible dose for the shortest possible duration necessary to relieve symptoms. In patients requiring longer-term treatment, consideration should be given to prescribing short courses on an as-required basis where appropriate. In patients requiring long-term treatment, monitoring of magnesium levels should be considered.

What drug interactions are important?

By increasing gastric pH, antacids and antisecretory medicines may affect the stability of enteric-coated formulations. These may break down at increased pH, resulting in the release of the medicine higher in the GI tract than was intended, with a resulting reduction in absorption. The absorption of other medicines may be dependent upon the acidic environment in the stomach, and an increase in pH can result in a subsequent reduction in absorption (e.g. ketoconazole).

Antacids. Metal ions present in antacid preparations may combine with certain medicines, resulting in the formation of insoluble compounds, which are poorly absorbed. These include some antibiotics (e.g. quinolones and tetracyclines) and penicillamine. Where possible, antacids should be administered at separate times to other medicines to avoid effects on absorption.

H_2RAs. Cimetidine is an inhibitor of a number of cytochrome P450 isoenzymes, which can result in a reduction in the metabolism of other medicines and a subsequent increase their plasma levels. This can be particularly problematic for medicines with a narrow therapeutic range such as phenytoin and theophylline, where toxicity may occur. For this reason, cimetidine is now rarely used in clinical practice.

PPIs. Particular care should be taken with the use of certain medicines used for the treatment of HIV infection.

Discontinuing treatment

When discontinuing PPIs, the dose should normally be reduced gradually before stopping to minimise the risk of rebound acid secretion and recurrence of symptoms. This may be more problematic following discontinuation after prolonged use.

35 Laxatives

Commonly used examples

The laxatives used to treat constipation are classified into four main categories, which assist with understanding the mechanism of action of the drug:

bulk-forming laxatives, e.g. ispaghula husk (Fybogel®), methylcellulose (Celevac®), and sterculia (Normacol and Normacol plus®)
faecal softeners, e.g. arachis oil, docusate sodium (Dioctyl®), and liquid paraffin
osmotic laxatives, e.g. lactulose, macrogol compound preparations (Movicol®), magnesium hydroxide, and sodium acid phosphate with sodium phosphate (Fleet enemas®)
stimulant laxatives, e.g. bisacodyl (Dulco-lax®), co-danthramer, co-danthrusate, glycerol, senna, and sodium picosulphate.

In addition to the groups listed above there are a number of medications that are used to manage specific cases of constipation that do not fall into the categories listed above:

linaclotide (Constella®)
lubiprostone (Amitiza®)
opioid receptor antagonists, e.g. methylnaltrexone bromide and naloxegol (Moventig®)
prucalopride (Resolor®).

Are these drugs all the same?

Laxatives all help to facilitate the passage of stools. However, different drugs achieve this in different ways.

What are these drugs used to treat?

All of these medications are used to treat constipation, although some may be reserved for certain situations. Prucalopride is only indicated for symptomatic treatment of chronic constipation in adults in whom other laxatives have failed to provide adequate relief.

Some have specific additional uses. Osmotic laxatives such as the Macrogol preparations (e.g. Movicol and Klean-Prep®) are also used for bowel cleansing, sometimes referred to as 'bowel prep'. This is the cleansing of faeces from the colon prior to a procedure such as a colonoscopy or prior to bowel surgery. Lactulose is used to treat hepatic encephalopathy, which can result from an increase in ammonium compounds in the bodies of patients with hepatic impairment. Lactulose inhibits the production of ammonia by gut bacteria (therefore reducing the absorption of ammonia from the gut) and increases its transit through the bowel. This prevents build-up of ammonia in the gut and subsequently in the blood, reducing the signs and symptoms of hepatic encephalopathy.

Rapid Medicines Management for Healthcare Professionals, First Edition. Paul Deslandes, Simon Young and Ben Pitcher.
© 2020 John Wiley & Sons Ltd. Published 2020 by John Wiley & Sons Ltd.

What do these drugs do?

The mechanism of action of bulk-forming laxatives is to increase faecal bulk. They are mainly comprised of non-absorbable fibre and carbohydrate. Their bulking up of faeces stimulates peristaltic action in the large intestine and this facilitates the passage of stools. As this group of medicines essentially emulates the role of dietary fibre, it may take several days for resolution of constipation. Maintaining an appropriate fluid intake is important with this group of medicines.

Faecal softeners 'soften' the stool by allowing fluid and fats to easily penetrate into it. The increase in fat and water content facilitates passage of the stool. Some members of this group also lubricate the stool and stimulate bowel movements.

Osmotic laxatives increase the water present in the large intestine. This increases stool volume, stimulates peristalsis, and facilitates stool passage. Medications such as lactulose often take two to three days to relieve constipation.

Stimulant laxatives act by directly stimulating the gut and increasing intestinal motility. The action of these medications is fairly quick. For example, if senna is dosed in the evening or at night, the passage of a stool usually occurs the following morning.

Linaclotide is specifically indicated for the treatment of constipation associated with irritable bowel syndrome. It stimulates the guanylate cyclase receptors on the luminal surface of the gastrointestinal epithelium. It emulates the activity of the endogenous guanylin peptides, which increases gastrointestinal transit in the gut but also have the added benefit of reducing visceral pain. Lubiprostone is an autacoid chloride channel activator. By specifically activating a chloride channel in the gut it increases fluid secretion in the intestine and increases the motility of the intestine. It is licenced for use in chronic idiopathic constipation when other interventions have not succeeded. Opioid receptor antagonists such as methylnaltrexone bromide are *peripheral* opioid antagonists. They antagonise the constipating effect of opioid analgesics. They do not adversely affect the analgesic activity of the opioids. Prucalopride is a selective, high-affinity 5-HT$_4$ receptor agonist. Agonism of this receptor in the gastrointestinal tract results in a prokinetic effect, which explains its laxative effect.

How are these drugs given?

The bulk-forming laxatives are given orally and their administration is required on a regular basis in order to restore and sustain bowel function. They are often presented as granules or sachets that need to be mixed with water before administration. Faecal softeners are dosed either orally or rectally (as enemas or suppositories) depending upon the product. Osmotic laxatives are given orally as liquids or as powders that need to be mixed to form a solution. For bowel prep, larger volumes of liquid are used for a shorter duration when compared with the management of constipation. Stimulant laxatives such as senna are typically given orally but stimulants are also available as rectally dosed preparations.

The nature of the constipation will dictate the duration of use of the product.

Linaclotide, lubiprostone, naloxegol, and prucalopride are available as oral dosage forms. Methylnaltrexone bromide is available as a solution for subcutaneous action.

What are the notable adverse effects to look out for?

Notable adverse effects include abdominal discomfort, distension, pain, bloating, and abdominal cramps. Nausea and gastrointestinal discomfort are also reported. Electrolyte disturbance can occur with excessive use. Co-danthramer and co-danthrusate may colour the urine red and have been associated with carcinogenicity. Their use is limited to terminally ill patients.

What needs to be monitored?

Monitoring of the bowel habit and fluid consumption of the patient are usually the most pertinent indicators of the efficacious and safe use of the medications.

What drug interactions are important?

None of note.

Other considerations

Constipation is a frequently encountered side effect of medication. Anticholinergic drugs, the opioids, and the anti-psychotic clozapine are some important examples. These examples illustrate where the efficacy of medications and their adverse effects have to be balanced and adequately managed to avoid constipation and its more serious sequelae.

Misuse of laxatives can occur, particularly in the context of certain eating disorders or if treatment is not reviewed and discontinued after symptoms have resolved.

Combination products of the four main groups are also available, e.g. senna and ispa-ghula husk as a single formulation.

36 Drugs Acting on the Renin Angiotensin System

Commonly used examples

Angiotensin converting enzyme (ACE) inhibitors. Ramipril, lisinopril, captopril, enalapril.
Angiotensin-II receptor antagonists, also called angiotensin receptor blockers. Losartan, candesartan, irbesartan, valsartan.

Are these drugs all the same?

No. Whilst the aim of all of these drugs is to prevent the action of angiotensin-II, their mechanisms of action are quite different. As such, their side effect profiles can also be quite different.

What are these drugs used to treat?

Both ACE inhibitors and angiotensin-II receptor antagonists are most commonly used to treat hypertension and heart failure.

What do these drugs do?

The renin–angiotensin system is part of the body's own control mechanism for blood pressure. In response to a drop in blood pressure, the body initiates a series of reactions, which ultimately produce the signalling molecule angiotensin-II. This has multiple actions on many different tissues and organs bringing about increases in blood pressure through vasoconstriction and increased fluid retention. Inhibiting the production or action of angiotensin-II will prevent these effects from occurring, and will therefore ameliorate rises in blood pressure and reduce cardiac workload.

What's the difference between ACE inhibitors and Angiotensin-II receptor antagonists?

Angiotensin-II is produced when needed by a multistage process facilitated by enzymes. One key enzyme that is responsible for converting the inactive precursor, angiotensin-I, into the active hormone angiotensin-II is ACE. ACE inhibitors stop this enzyme from working and thereby prevent angiotensin-II from being produced. This therefore prevents the subsequent actions of angiotensin-II from occurring.

The effects of angiotensin-II in various tissues are mediated through it binding to angiotensin-II receptors. Angiotensin-II antagonists block this receptor and prevent the angiotensin-II from having an effect.

Rapid Medicines Management for Healthcare Professionals, First Edition. Paul Deslandes, Simon Young and Ben Pitcher.
© 2020 John Wiley & Sons Ltd. Published 2020 by John Wiley & Sons Ltd.

How are these drugs given?

These agents are given orally in tablet form, usually once or twice a day on a long-term basis for the management of cardiovascular disease.

Dosing

At the start of treatment, ACE inhibitors can have a pronounced effect and should therefore be introduced gradually, particularly in patients receiving diuretics and those with heart failure and certain other co-morbidities.

What are the notable adverse effects to look out for?

Some of the adverse effects associated with these medicines are common to both ACE inhibitors and angiotensin-II receptor antagonists and are extensions of their main action. However, ACE inhibitors are generally considered to cause more problematic adverse effects. Their effects on blood pressure can be pronounced and cause symptomatic hypotension (particularly if given in conjunction with other antihypertensives).

Due to effects on renal blood flow, these medicines can lead to renal impairment and acute kidney injury (AKI). By interfering with the body's retention of fluids there is a resulting impact on electrolytes. In particular, these medicines are known to increase levels of potassium. This should be considered if the patient is receiving any other medication that might cause hyperkalaemia (such as spironolactone and other potassium-sparing diuretics).

The therapeutic effects of ACE inhibitors are related to the inhibition of angiotensin-II synthesis. However, this is not the only thing that ACE does. ACE is also involved in the deactivation of bradykinin (an inflammatory mediator). This means that whilst ACE inhibitors prevent the production of angiotensin-II, they also cause an accumulation of bradykinin. This is believed to cause two notable adverse effects that affect some patients. A build-up of bradykinin in the lungs is associated with a dry irritating cough. This can be quite distracting for patients and is a common reason for treatment discontinuation. Excessive build-up of bradykinin is also believed to cause angioedema. This swelling of the tongue and throat can appear similar to anaphylaxis and has the potential to be fatal. The incidence of this is common enough for it to be colloquially referred to as 'Lisinopril tongue'.

ACE inhibitors should be avoided in pregnancy due to the risks of adverse effects (including teratogenesis) in the developing foetus.

How can the adverse effects be minimised?

As angiotensin-II receptor antagonists have no direct action on ACE, they do not trigger increased levels of bradykinin. As such, they do not tend to cause a dry cough or angioedema. This makes them good alternatives for patients who are experiencing these problematic side effects of ACE inhibitors. Angioedema is particularly common in patients of Afro-Caribbean ethnicity, and angiotensin-II receptor antagonists are preferred in this patient group. It is important to note, however, that angioedema has been reported following use of angiotensin receptor antagonists, although the mechanism for this is not fully understood.

What needs to be monitored?

As these drugs can have a pronounced effect on blood pressure it is important that this is monitored. This is especially true during early treatment. ACE inhibitors and angiotensin-II receptor antagonists are known to cause hyperkalaemia and impaired renal function, therefore serum potassium levels and renal function should be monitored after initiation, dose changes and on an ongoing basis.

What drug interactions are important?

As ACE inhibitors can cause retention of potassium they should be used with caution with potassium supplements and other drugs that cause an increase in serum potassium, such potassium-sparing diuretics (e.g. spironolactone). Drugs acting on different aspects of the renin–angiotensin system (i.e. ACE inhibitors, angiotensin-II receptor antagonists. and aliskiren) should not be used in combination unless under specialist supervision. Non-steroidal anti-inflammatory drugs (e.g. ibuprofen and naproxen) can increase the risk of renal impairment. Lithium levels can be increased by both ACE inhibitors and angiotensin-II receptor antagonists, with the potential to cause toxicity.

37 Beta-Blockers

Beta-blockers are also known as beta-adrenoceptor blocking drugs or beta-adrenoceptor antagonists.

Commonly used examples
Atenolol, bisoprolol, propranolol, carvedilol, oxprenolol, sotalol, timolol.

Are these drugs all the same?
The basic pharmacology of these drugs is broadly similar. They all bind to beta-adrenergic receptors, preventing adrenaline or noradrenaline from binding and thereby preventing the increase in cardiac workload and blood pressure that this would cause. The differences come from how selective they are (do they block adrenergic receptors elsewhere in the body, causing side effects) or whether they have any intrinsic sympathomimetic activity (acting as partial agonists at the receptor) and thereby cause a milder response. Beta-blockers also vary in their lipid solubility. This results in different pharmacokinetic properties, with the more lipid-soluble drugs (e.g. metoprolol and propranolol) being more able to cross the blood–brain barrier and being metabolised in the liver.

What are these drugs used to treat?
Beta-blockers reduce the activity of the heart. As a result, they lower blood pressure and are used in the treatment of hypertension. They can also be used to treat angina (lower cardiac workload means lower cardiac oxygen requirements) and heart failure (e.g. bisoprolol, carvedilol, and nebivolol). The increase in heart rate associated with the action of the sympathetic nervous system (SNS) can make the heart more prone to abnormal rhythms. By inhibiting this effect, beta-blockers reduce the incidence of some arrhythmias and are therefore used as antiarrhythmic agents. Beta-blockers can also be administered as eye drops in the management of certain types of glaucoma.

What do these drugs do?
One of the main mechanisms the body has for controlling its physiological functions is the autonomic nervous system. The SNS forms part of this mechanism, and uses adrenaline and noradrenaline as its chemical signalling molecules. These chemical messengers bind to adrenoceptors in different organs and tissues to elicit responses throughout the body. There are different subsets of adrenoceptors, which are found on different organs and tissues, and mediate different physiological effects. The beta-1 receptor is found on the heart, and when stimulated by adrenaline or noradrenaline increases heart rate and strength of contraction, increasing cardiac output and therefore blood

Rapid Medicines Management for Healthcare Professionals, First Edition. Paul Deslandes, Simon Young and Ben Pitcher.
© 2020 John Wiley & Sons Ltd. Published 2020 by John Wiley & Sons Ltd.

pressure. Beta-blockers act as antagonists at the beta-1 receptor, essentially preventing the SNS from raising (or maintaining) a high blood pressure.

Beta-receptors are also present in other organs and tissues, including the brain, eye, airways, and vascular system. Receptors at these sites may include the beta-2 type receptors, but most beta-blockers can have an effect at these receptors as well as those in the heart. Blocking receptors in other tissues may result in therapeutic effects such as in the treatment of anxiety (e.g. propranolol) and glaucoma or adverse effects such as bronchoconstriction or vasoconstriction.

How are these drugs given?

Beta-blockers may be given orally (in tablet or liquid form), usually on a long-term basis for the management of cardiac disorders. Esmolol and labetalol can be given intravenously on a short-term basis for hypertension or arrhythmia. Eye drops (e.g. betaxolol, carteolol, timolol) are usually given twice a day on a long-term basis for the management of open angle glaucoma.

What are the notable adverse effects to look out for?

Adverse effects are associated with the effects of the medication on the heart and vascular system. Bradycardia, symptomatic hypotension, and cold peripheries are common.

Whilst beta-blockers block beta-1 receptors, they can also have an effect on other receptor subtypes, particularly beta-2 receptors. When stimulated beta-2 receptors cause bronchodilation, so blocking them can trigger bronchospasm. Due to this beta-blockers are contraindicated in asthma.

How can the adverse effects be minimised?

Side effects can only really be managed rather than reduced. Notable side effects such as postural hypertension can be affected by the choice of beta-blocker. Some beta-blockers are referred to as partial agonists. They bind to the beta-1 receptors and produce a moderate response, which means they are in fact agonists. However, because they produce a smaller response than the endogenous agonist (adrenaline/noradrenaline) they still reduce the activity of the heart and therefore blood pressure. They are arguably less effective but the adverse effects are milder, for example vasoconstriction may be reduced.

Similarly, some beta-blockers are more selective (have more of an effect) on beta-1 receptors (e.g. atenolol and bisoprolol) and therefore have fewer adverse effects on the airways. Others (e.g. propranolol and timolol) are more selective for beta-2 receptors and are more likely to cause bronchoconstriction.

What drug interactions are important?

Beta-blockers can have some notable interactions with other cardiac drugs, particularly with drugs that cause bradycardia such as rate-limiting calcium channel blockers (especially verapamil). Lipid-soluble beta-blockers undergo metabolism by cytochrome P450 enzymes in the liver, and can interact with inducers (e.g. carbamazepine) and inhibitors (e.g. paroxetine) of these enzymes.

Discontinuing treatment

The body tends to adapt to changes imposed by drugs. In response to the reduced level of SNS stimulation (resulting from the use of beta-blockers), the number of beta-1 adrenoceptors present on cardiac cells will be up-regulated (increased). This causes little difficulty whilst the patient is receiving treatment and the receptors are blocked. However, if the beta-blocker is abruptly stopped, the increased number of receptors will trigger a greater response from endogenous adrenaline and noradrenaline, resulting in rebound hypertension. Due to this beta-blockers should not be stopped abruptly, but instead the dose titrated down gradually.

38 Diuretics

Commonly used examples

Loop diuretics
  Furosemide
  Torasemide
  Bumetanide
Thiazides
  Bendroflumethiazide
  Indapamide
Potassium sparing
  Spironolactone
  Eplerenone
  Amiloride hydrochloride

Are these drugs all the same?

Diuretic drugs achieve their effects by subtly different means. Most of the more widely used diuretics (loop diuretics, thiazides, and potassium-sparing diuretics) inhibit the transport of electrolytes out of the renal tubule. By preventing the removal of the electrolytes they reduce the osmotic gradient and prevent the reabsorption of water by the kidney. They also prevent the reabsorption of the electrolyte, resulting in its loss from the body in the urine. Different diuretics can inhibit the reabsorption of different electrolytes; this means that whilst they all increase urine output they have different impacts on electrolyte balance and blood chemistry.

What are these drugs used to treat?

Typically, the increased diuresis is intended to remove excess fluid from the body. The reduction in the amount of water in the blood will reduce the circulating volume and lower blood pressure. The reduced water content in the blood will also help shift fluid from other tissues back into the blood, reducing oedema. Diuretics are therefore widely used in the treatment of hypertension and conditions such as heart failure. They can even be used in emergencies such as pulmonary oedema.

In some rarer circumstances a diuretic may be used to specifically facilitate the loss of a given electrolyte from the body. Acetazolamide is a carbonic anhydrase inhibitor, essentially preventing the reabsorption of bicarbonate ions. Whilst this will have the effect of increasing urine output, it is usually given to facilitate the loss of bicarbonate ions and correct a base excess.

Rapid Medicines Management for Healthcare Professionals, First Edition. Paul Deslandes, Simon Young and Ben Pitcher.
© 2020 John Wiley & Sons Ltd. Published 2020 by John Wiley & Sons Ltd.

What do these drugs do?

Urine formation within the nephron has three major components: filtration, reabsorption, and secretion. In the filtration phase, blood is forced through the glomerulus under high pressure, squeezing water and electrolytes into the Bowman's capsule and into the tubule. Most of the water will then need to be reabsorbed. This achieved by a process of transporting electrolytes out of the tubule, creating an osmotic gradient and allowing the water to move out of the tubule and back into the blood supply. This concept is often described by the simplified 'where the salt goes the water follows'.

Diuretics reduce the osmotic gradient between the tubule and the surrounding tissue, and therefore reduce the amount of water reabsorbed, resulting in more urine being produced.

What's the difference between loop diuretics, thiazides, and potassium-sparing diuretics?

Loop diuretics are powerful and fast acting, taking effect within one hour of administration. They cause the loss of sodium and potassium ions (the loss of potassium is the most likely cause of adverse events or interference with the actions of other medications).

Thiazides are slower to act but their effects last for a longer period, cause loss of sodium and potassium ions, but tend to have less severe effects on blood chemistry, which makes them a more typical choice for long-term treatment.

Potassium-sparing diuretics act in one of two ways. First, they disrupt the action of the endogenous hormone aldosterone. Aldosterone normally facilitates the movement of sodium and potassium ions into and out of the tubule, causing water to be reabsorbed. Drugs like spironolactone and eplerenone directly block the aldosterone receptor, negating its effect. Second, the potassium-sparing diuretic amiloride blocks ion channels, preventing the resorption of sodium. This results in a loss of sodium but an increased retention of potassium. The effect means they are sometimes used in conjunction with loop diuretics, the potassium-sparing effects of amiloride counteracts the "potassium-losing" effects of the loop diuretic.

How are these drugs given?

For the majority of patients, diuretics will be given in tablet form. However, in acute and critically ill patients, diuretics may be given intravenously. They are also licensed for intramuscular administration but this is rarely seen.

What are the notable adverse effects to look out for?

All diuretics will increase urine output. However, it is important to consider how the patient will experience this. Unless the patient is catheterised, they will experience increased frequency and urgency of urination. If the patient has reduced mobility, problems with sight or is in unfamiliar circumstances this can lead to incontinence or falls. Some patients attempt to address this issue themselves by reducing their own fluid intake. This can unfortunately lead to dehydration and urinary tract infections.

As discussed above the diuretics' mechanism of action will often result in the additional loss of electrolytes. This can cause a deranged blood chemistry. Loop diuretics (such as furosemide) are often associated with hypokalaemia, while potassium-sparing diuretics are associated with hyperkalaemia.

The net loss of water from the blood can have an effect of increasing the relative concentrations of the solutes in blood. There have been reports of hyperglycaemia in diabetics and hyperuricemia leading to gout as a result of diuretic use.

Aldosterone antagonists such as spironolactone act by blocking the aldosterone receptor. However, they are capable of blocking the receptors of other similarly structured hormones such as androgens. This anti-androgenic effect can cause problems such as menstrual disturbances or gynecomastia. Eplerenone is also an aldosterone antagonist but is more selective and therefore does not cause the same anti-androgenic side effects.

If furosemide is administered in an acute or critical situation, it may be administered intravenously. If the furosemide is injected too quickly it can cause tinnitus, therefore it should be administered slowly (less than $4\,mg\,min^{-1}$ or even slower in patients with renal failure).

How can the adverse effects be minimised?

The impact of diuretics on urinary frequency and urgency can be reduced to certain degree by timing the dose with what best suits the patient.

What needs to be monitored?

Electrolytes may need to be checked before commencing and whilst diuretics are being used. Renal function can be impacted by diuretic use and therefore may need to be monitored. In more acute circumstances it may often be necessary to monitor urine output in order to ascertain the effectiveness of the treatment. Due to the effect of reducing circulating volume patients' blood pressure may also need to be monitored, especially when first started on diuretics.

What drug interactions are important?

Most notable interactions are associated with the disruption of electrolytes. The hypokalaemia attributed to loop diuretics can increase the toxicity of digoxin and other cardiac drugs. Potassium-sparing diuretics may cause issues if they are taken with other agents that cause hyperkalaemia, such as angiotensin converting enzyme inhibitors (see Chapter 36) or potassium supplements.

Diuretics (particularly thiazides) can result in retention of lithium, with increased plasma levels and the potential for lithium toxicity.

Non-steroidal anti-inflammatory drugs (NSAIDs) can cause sodium and water retention, and may worsen congestive heart failure. Combined use of NSAIDs and diuretics may increase the risk of renal impairment and acute kidney injury, and may also reduce the effectiveness of diuretics.

39 Anticoagulants

Commonly used examples

Coumarins
  Warfarin
Direct oral anticoagulants (DOACs)
  Thrombin inhibitor – dabigatran
  Factor Xa inhibitors – apixaban, edoxaban, rivaroxaban
Heparins
  Unfractionated heparin
  Low molecular weight heparins: dalteparin, enoxaparin

Are these drugs all the same?

Whilst all anticoagulants achieve the same general outcome, preventing the formation of clots (thrombi), there are several distinct groups of anticoagulants. The different groups have different mechanisms of action, different routes of administration, and different monitoring requirements. It is important to understand these differences to ensure effective management of these medicines. The main groups to be aware of are coumarins, heparins, and DOACs.

Another similar group are the antiplatelet drugs. These reduce platelet aggregation and are also used to prevent the formation of clots. Antiplatelet drugs are discussed in Chapter 40.

What are these drugs used to treat?

Most anticoagulants are used prophylactically to prevent the development of clots. Whilst the ability of the blood to clot is an important part of the body's haemostatic processes and is essential for normal healing of cuts and wounds, if a clot forms in the bloodstream it can have dire consequences. If blood flow slows and the blood becomes static (such as in the leg veins of an immobile patient or in the atria of patient with atrial fibrillation) the blood can begin to coagulate and form thrombi. These thrombi can block blood vessels and prevent the flow of blood, which can precipitate serious problems such as strokes, myocardial infarctions, and pulmonary embolisms.

Whilst anticoagulants are most commonly used prophylactically, they can also be used as part of the treatment for patients who have had a thrombotic event.

What do these drugs do?

The coagulation of blood is a complex multistage process (often referred to as the coagulation cascade). This process is a chain reaction, where clotting factors are activated by tissue injury and activate the next set of clotting factors in the cascade, which in turn activate the

Rapid Medicines Management for Healthcare Professionals, First Edition. Paul Deslandes, Simon Young and Ben Pitcher.
© 2020 John Wiley & Sons Ltd. Published 2020 by John Wiley & Sons Ltd.

next set. This chain reaction continues until the final stage, where fibrinogen is converted into fibrin and a stable clot is formed. Anticoagulants are used to disrupt this cascade and prevent the formation of the clot.

What's the difference between different types?

Coumarins include the most commonly used anticoagulant, warfarin. They are used as long-term prophylaxis in patients who have an ongoing risk of thrombosis. These drugs interfere with the coagulation cascade by inhibiting a key enzyme (vitamin K epoxide reductase), which uses vitamin K to facilitate the activation of various coagulation factors within the coagulation cascade. As these drugs prevent the utilisation of vitamin K, they are sometimes referred to as vitamin K antagonists. However, this is not a truly accurate description of their mechanism of action.

DOACs are newer agents (they are sometime called novel oral anticoagulants), which inhibit specific coagulation factors within the coagulation cascade. Most of the drugs inhibit factor Xa, although dabigatran inhibits the action of thrombin. DOACs are growing in popularity, in part because they do not require international normalised ratio (INR) monitoring (see below).

Heparins are more commonly used in hospitals and may be used for short-term anticoagulation for patients in acute circumstances (such as following surgery). Heparin enhances the activity of antithrombin, which is responsible for deactivating thrombin. Normally antithrombin is responsible for keeping the coagulation cascade in check and preventing excessive coagulation. By enhancing the action of antithrombin, heparin is able to prevent a thrombus from forming. Whilst we typically associate heparins with prophylaxis they can also be given to patients who have a thrombus. However, this is not the same as thrombolysis, where drugs are given to specifically break down an existing clot.

Heparins are formed of polysaccharide chains of differing lengths. Unfractionated heparin is a solution that contains all the different lengths mixed together. Unfractionated heparin is potent but has a short duration of action and has an increased risk of adverse effects. It is generally only used in hospitals with critically ill patients. Low molecular weight heparins (LMWHs) are solutions of just the shorter polysaccharide chains. These tend to be longer acting (allowing once a day dosing) and more 'gentle', resulting in fewer adverse effects. Enoxaparin is a commonly used LMWH.

How are these drugs given?

Coumarins and DOACs are typically administered orally in tablet form. Heparins must be given parenterally, most commonly in the form of pre-filled subcutaneous injections.

Dosing

Different patients will have notably different responses to warfarin. This means that the dose required to achieve the desired level of anticoagulation (as measured by INR – see below) can vary considerably. The dose can be titrated up or down until the desired level of anticoagulation is achieved. This means that two patients with the same condition (e.g. atrial fibrillation) may be prescribed totally different doses of warfarin, with the intention of achieving the same level of anticoagulation.

DOACs are more predictable in their action and therefore tend to have more standardised doses given once or twice a day. Their effects are not as long lasting as those of warfarin and compliance with treatment is particularly important. Dosages may need to be reduced in patients with renal impairment.

Heparins can have set doses for different conditions, but they are commonly calculated according to weight (e.g. 1 mg/kg or 1.5 mg/kg). This can cause difficulties, as the LMWHs are usually available in pre-filled syringes, of which there are only a limited number of sizes.

If it is not possible to administer the dose prescribed, then it may be necessary to confirm with the prescriber how they wish to proceed. Your employer or work area may have a policy on how to manage this situation.

What are the notable adverse effects to look out for?

Whenever you are caring for patients taking anticoagulants, it is important to remember that coagulation is not an inherently bad thing. It is part of our body's haemostatic process intended to protect us from excessive blood loss in the case of injury. When anticoagulants are used to prevent excessive or unwanted clotting, we inevitably place the patient at increased risk of bleeding and bruising. If an anticoagulated patient experiences an injury (such as a fall) we must be particularly careful about potential bleeds or haematomas, particularly if the patient has hit their head.

Heparin is noted for its potential to cause thrombocytopenia (termed heparin-induced thrombocytopenia or HIT). This is more of a risk when using unfractionated heparin rather than LMWH.

How can the adverse effects be minimised?

The risk of bleeding can be reduced by ensuring that the INR is within the desired range and that the patient is not over-treated.

What needs to be monitored?

To achieve appropriate levels of coagulation, we need to be able to measure the relative ability of the blood to clot. This is usually done using one of two measures, either INR or activated thromboplastin (APTT).

INR stands for the international normalised ratio and is a representation of proportionally how long it will take blood to clot compared to 'normal' blood (based on the time taken for specific part of the coagulation cascade to occur). If the INR is 2 it means the blood will take twice as long to clot. If the INR is 3 then it will take three times as long to clot and so on. INR is notably used to assess the action of warfarin. A patient prescribed warfarin will be given a target INR and the dose will be titrated up and down to try and achieve this target. This means that the patient will probably need regular blood tests to ensure their dosing is correct. DOACs tend to have a more consistent level of activity, however monitoring of renal function is important.

APTT is a measure of the time take for an alternative part of the coagulation cascade (to that measured by INR) to occur. APTT can be represented as the number of seconds or as a ratio. The APTT ratio is more useful for assessing the effect of unfractionated heparin.

What drug interactions are important?

Any drug that further reduces the ability of the blood to clot should be used with care, as the cumulative effect can cause increased risk of bleeding. Examples include non-steroidal anti-inflammatory drugs and selective serotonin reuptake inhibitors.

Warfarin is associated with a number of drug interactions, which may result in an increased or decreased therapeutic effect. It should always be remembered that these interactions can occur with non-prescribed drugs like aspirin or ibuprofen, or even with foodstuffs like cabbage, cranberry juice, and alcoholic beverages. It is prudent to check the British National Formulary for any potential interactions.

The effects of DOACs can be influenced by cytochrome P450 enzyme inducers and inhibitors, and before administering co-prescribed medicines interactions should be considered.

Reversal agents

As coagulation is an important physiological process, it may be necessary to reverse the action of an anticoagulant in the event that a patient's INR is too high, or after a traumatic injury or if they need surgery. Different anticoagulants can be reversed using different agents.

It can be possible to restore a patient's ability to clot by infusing blood products or replacing specific clotting factors. As discussed above, warfarin acts by inhibiting the utilisation of vitamin K. Warfarin can therefore be reversed by giving the patient vitamin K. Heparin can be reversed using the drug protamine. This chemically reacts with the heparin, binding to it and rendering it inactive. DOACs have limited options for reversal. Dabigatran can be reversed using idarucizumab, a humanised monoclonal antibody that binds to dabigatran and prevents it from exerting its effect. Andexanet alfa is a reversal agent for factor Xa inhibitors. However, at the time of writing it did not have marketing authorisation in the UK.

40 Antiplatelets

Commonly used examples
Aspirin
Clopidogrel
Dipyridamole

Are these drugs all the same?
Whilst all antiplatelet drugs reduce the ability of platelets to aggregate and form a clot, they achieve this by different pharmacological mechanisms. As such, different antiplatelet drugs may be used for different conditions and will have different side effects and contraindications.

What are these drugs used to treat?
Antiplatelet drugs are used to prevent the formation of clots. The formation of clots is, of course, a vital part of haemostasis and is in itself not a harmful process. However, in certain circumstances clots (thrombi) can form in the blood and can block the flow of blood to tissues and organs. These thrombi can be the cause of serious and potentially life-threatening conditions such as myocardial infarctions, strokes, and pulmonary embolisms. Antiplatelets are therefore not so much a treatment for these conditions but a prophylactic, attempting to prevent them from occurring.

Antiplatelet drugs are commonly prescribed in circumstances where a patient has a risk of thrombosis such as atrial fibrillation or has a history of thrombosis. For example, clopidogrel is commonly used specifically used to prevent further thrombotic events in patients who have suffered a stroke or myocardial infarction.

What do these drugs do?
All antiplatelet drugs work by preventing the activation of platelets (thrombocytes), thereby preventing platelet aggregation and the formation of a clot. However, the different antiplatelet drugs achieve this by disrupting the normal function of the platelets in different ways.

Antiplatelet drugs may sometimes be referred to as 'blood thinners'. Whilst this term is commonly used it is not accurate. Antiplatelet drugs do not in fact dilute or reduce the viscosity of the blood.

What's the difference between different types?
Aspirin is one of the best known antiplatelet drugs. Although historically it may have been associated with its actions as an analgesic and antipyretic, it is now more commonly used an antiplatelet. Aspirin inhibits the cyclooxygenase (COX) enzymes which are responsible

Rapid Medicines Management for Healthcare Professionals, First Edition. Paul Deslandes, Simon Young and Ben Pitcher.
© 2020 John Wiley & Sons Ltd. Published 2020 by John Wiley & Sons Ltd.

for synthesising numerous chemical messengers such as prostaglandins and prostacyclins. It is the broad range of substances that are produced by COX (and whose synthesis is inhibited by aspirin) that account for aspirin's numerous actions and side effects. Within the thrombocyte, COX is responsible for producing thromboxane, a key factor in cell activation. Inhibiting COX prevents the production of thromboxane and therefore prevents the activation and aggregation of platelets. It is this same action which accounts for the increased risk of bleeding and bruising seen with other COX inhibitors (e.g. ibuprofen).

Clopidogrel blocks ADP receptors on the platelet, which plays an important role in platelet activation and aggregation. Clopidogrel is a prodrug, an inactive chemical that is converted into the active form by liver enzymes. Any variance in the activity of these enzymes can influence the effectiveness of the drug. This can be caused by genetic variation or the action of other drugs. Some newer drugs (ticagrelor) work in the same way as clopidogrel but are not prodrugs and therefore avoid this potential variation in activity.

Dipyridamole inhibits the uptake of adenosine into the platelets, resulting in reduced ability to aggregate and form a clot.

How are these drugs given?
Most antiplatelet drugs are given orally, typically in tablet form. Oral suspensions and liquids are available for some medications.

Dosing
Dosing for antiplatelet drugs is usually a standard dose taken once daily.

Aspirin. It is important to note that with regard to aspirin the dose used for its antiplatelet action (75 mg once a day) is significantly lower than that used for analgesia (300–900 mg every 4–6 hours). The 75 mg tablets are sometimes referred to as 'mini aspirin' 'daily aspirin', or even 'baby aspirin'.

What are some notable adverse effects to look out for?
Antiplatelet drugs are intended to reduce the ability of the blood to form clots. As a result, patients who take them are at increased risk of bruising and bleeding.

Aspirin, like other COX inhibitors, can cause gastric irritation. Even though the dose is quite small, the fact that it is taken daily for extended periods of time can lead to a cumulative damage that may result in gastric ulceration. Because of this it is recommended that aspirin should only be taken as a prophylactic if there is an identified risk of thrombosis.

How can the adverse effects be minimised?
The gastric irritation caused by aspirin can be minimised by ensuring that it is taken with food.

What needs to be monitored?
As antiplatelet drugs affect clotting in a different way to anticoagulants such as warfarin and heparin, their effects are not measured using the international normalised ratio or activated partial thromboplastin time. However, if these are elevated the administered antiplatelet drugs may place the patient at increased risk of bleeding.

What drug interactions are important?

If antiplatelet drugs are combined with any other agent known to reduce clotting (such as anticoagulants) then there is a significant increased risk of bleeding and bruising. As such they should be generally avoided. It should also be noted that drugs such as non-steroidal anti-inflammatory drugs (NSAIDs) and selective serotonin reuptake inhibitors can inhibit platelet aggregation and may increase the risk of bleeding.

Aspirin can cause gastric irritation and should therefore be used with caution with other drugs that can cause gastric irritation such as corticosteroids and other NSAIDs.

Clopidogrel's action may be influenced by agents that affect its bioconversion in the liver. This can include interaction with drugs (e.g. fluconazole and fluoxetine) and even some foodstuffs (e.g. grapefruit juice).

A full list of interactions can be found in the *British National Formulary*.

41 Inotropes

Commonly used examples

Adrenaline
Dobutamine
Dopamine
Noradrenaline

Are these drugs all the same?

Whilst all inotropes are used to achieve the same overall effect, an increase in blood pressure, there are some subtle differences as to how they achieve this, which dictates why different inotropes are be used in different circumstances.

What are these drugs used to treat?

Inotropes are used to help boost blood pressure with the aim of restoring adequate perfusion of the organs and tissues. This can be necessary in patients whose cardiovascular system has been compromised. This may be due to damage to the heart itself (cardiogenic shock), a loss of circulating volume due to haemorrhage (haemorrhagic shock) or dehydration (hypovolaemic shock), or it can be caused by a systemic vasodilation such as that caused by a systemic infection (septic shock) or systemic allergic reaction (anaphylactic shock). In these cases, the underlying problems will need to be corrected if the patient has any hope of recovery, but inotropes can help to support the cardiovascular system and keep the patient alive until the underlying problems can be corrected.

What do these drugs do?

When considering the action of inotropes, it is helpful to consider how blood pressure is maintained. Blood pressure (BP) can be considered to be a product of cardiac output (CO) and peripheral vascular resistance (PVR):

$$BP = CO \times PVR$$

Cardiac output is itself the product of heart rate and stroke volume. Peripheral vascular resistance is a measure of the resistance to flow the blood experiences as it flows through the blood vessels. Whilst this is multifactorial, the most variable factor is the diameter of the blood vessel (the narrower the blood vessels the harder it is for blood to flow through). It is therefore possible to increase blood pressure by increasing cardiac output, by increasing peripheral vascular resistance (via vasoconstriction) or increasing both. The body homeostatically maintains blood pressure on a moment by moment basis, e.g. blood pressure

Rapid Medicines Management for Healthcare Professionals, First Edition. Paul Deslandes, Simon Young and Ben Pitcher.
© 2020 John Wiley & Sons Ltd. Published 2020 by John Wiley & Sons Ltd.

increases in response to a stimulus influencing the sympathetic nervous system using adrenaline (epinephrine) and noradrenaline. As these agents mimic or enhance the normal actions of the sympathetic nervous system, they are also called sympathomimetics.

What are the differences between different types?

Some inotropes are the same as the endogenous biochemicals utilised by the body; adrenaline and noradrenaline are two of the chemical messengers of the sympathetic nervous system and are used to raise blood pressure as part of normal homeostasis.

Dopamine is also produced naturally in the body. Although it is more commonly thought of as a neurotransmitter in the brain, it has a very similar structure to adrenaline and will stimulate adrenergic receptors. Other inotropes, such as dobutamine, are not found naturally in the body but are chemically synthesised molecules with a similar molecular structure to those produced endogenously.

All inotropes increase blood pressure, but how much of the increase that is due to increasing cardiac output and how much is due to increased vasoconstriction varies from drug to drug. Adrenaline, dopamine, and dobutamine have a greater effect on increasing cardiac output whilst noradrenaline is used more for its vasoconstrictor properties.

How are these drugs given?

Inotropes have a relatively short half-life of about 2–3 minutes. In order to maintain an appropriate blood pressure the only viable option is to deliver the drug by continuous infusion (usually using a form of syringe pump).

Important note

As the half-life of the drugs is relatively short, if the infusion is interrupted the patient's blood pressure may begin to drop quickly. To prevent this, it is essential to keep track of how much of the drug is left in the delivery device (and how soon it will run out) and prepare the replacement syringe in good time so that it can swapped with minimal disruption to the infusion.

Dosing

Due to the very precise titrations required, for some inotropes it is normal practice to calculate the infusion rate in terms of micrograms per kilogram per minute. Dosing rates will then be titrated up and down to keep the blood pressure within acceptable parameters (such as a target mean arterial pressure [MAP]).

What are the notable adverse effects to look out for?

Most side effects seen are extensions of the normal action of these drugs (e.g. tachycardia, anxiety), but some of these actions can become problematic if they become too pronounced.

Inotropes such as noradrenaline boost blood pressure by causing vasoconstriction and increased peripheral vascular resistance. This vasoconstriction can prevent adequate blood supply reaching peripheral tissues. This can cause tissue ischemia and even tissue death and necrosis around the site of infusion or in the periphery. Prolonged usage of vasoconstrictors can cause necrosis in the hands and fingers; they may become blackened and have to be amputated.

How can the adverse effects be minimised?

Inotropes are generally only used in critically ill patients, as such the side effects they cause may be seen as an unfortunate but unavoidable feature of the drug's use. Accurate formulation, dosing, and monitoring of therapy are the cornerstones of efficacious and safe use of inotropes.

What needs to be monitored?

Patients being administered inotropes will usually need continuous monitoring of the cardiovascular system. Inotropes are only typically seen in acute care areas such as accident and emergency and critical care where close monitoring of the patient is required.

What drug interactions are important?

Inotropes can have notable interactions with other agents that affect a patient's blood pressure. Notable examples of this include interactions with beta-blockers. Excessive hypertension can also be caused by the use of inotropes with drugs that interfere with the removal or deactivation of inotropes, such as tricyclic antidepressants or monoamine oxidase inhibitors.

Discontinuing treatment

Inotropes are typically reduced gradually, titrating the dose down with the aim of maintaining a suitable blood pressure. If they are withdrawn suddenly, the patient may become hypotensive.

42 Anti-anginals

Commonly used examples

Beta-blockers, e.g. acebutolol, atenolol, bisoprolol, carvedilol, metoprolol, nadolol, oxprenolol, propranolol, and timolol.

Calcium channel blockers, e.g. amlodipine, diltiazem, felodipine, nicardipine, nifedipine, and verapamil.

Ivabradine

Nicorandil

Nitrates, e.g. glyceryl trinitrate, isosorbide dinitrate, and isosorbide mononitrate.

Ranolazine

Are these drugs all the same?

Beta-blockers have many indications but in angina they reduce the workload of cardiac muscle and this improves exercise tolerance and relieves the symptoms of angina. Calcium channel blockers have a variety of indications: they cause vasodilation, reduce the work of the myocardium and slow cardiac conductance relieving angina symptoms. The nitrates are broken down into the vasodilator nitric oxide (NO), and increase blood and oxygen flow to the heart, reducing symptoms of angina. Ranolazine interferes with sodium currents but its exact mechanism of action in unknown.

What are these drugs used to treat?

This group of medications are used to prevent the onset of the symptoms of angina and/or to relieve the symptoms of angina.

What do these drugs do?

Beta-blockers, as their name suggests, block beta-receptors. These beta-receptors mediate the effects of sympathetic nervous system stimulants such as adrenaline. When beta-blockers bind to the receptor, they prevent the increased rate and force of cardiac contraction, selective vasoconstriction, and other effects of adrenaline that raise blood pressure. This, in turn, prevents the symptoms of angina.

The influx of calcium ions to the cells of the myocardium and the smooth muscle of the vasculature promotes constriction of these muscle tissues. This results in speedier conductance in cardiac tissue, increases the force and rate of contraction of the myocardium, and promotes vasoconstriction, resulting in increased effort on the part of the myocardium. Calcium channel blockers prevent the influx of calcium into cells and prevent the development of these effects. Ivabradine reduces heart rate by interfering with the pacemaker cells of the heart, slowing heart rate and allowing increased myocardial blood flow. Nicorandil

Rapid Medicines Management for Healthcare Professionals, First Edition. Paul Deslandes, Simon Young and Ben Pitcher.
© 2020 John Wiley & Sons Ltd. Published 2020 by John Wiley & Sons Ltd.

causes smooth muscle relaxation and coronary vasodilation by interfering with the activity of calcium in smooth muscle cells.

The endothelial cells of blood vessel walls produce a signalling molecule, NO. This compound promotes smooth muscle relaxation and allows the vessels to dilate. This causes increased blood flow through the vessel and, in angina, relieves the symptoms. The nitrates listed above are broken down to form NO and promote the relaxation of smooth muscle by the same pathways utilised by endogenous NO.

How are these drugs given?

Beta-blockers are taken orally to treat angina. They are usually dosed daily or twice daily according to the licensing and pharmacokinetics of the beta-blocker used (there is some variation, e.g. propranolol). They need to be taken regularly and not discontinued or withdrawn abruptly unless this is clinically indicated (see the section on other considerations).

Calcium channel blockers are also dosed orally (note that not all calcium channel blockers are licenced for use in the treatment of angina). The frequency of dosing, as with beta-blockers, is dependent on the individual drug and its formulation.

Ivabradine is available as tablets and it should be noted that it is used in adults in normal sinus rhythm and a heart rate equal to or greater than 70 bpm (in angina) – the criteria differ when ivabradine is used in heart failure.

Nicorandil is available as oral tablets. The medication is administered twice daily and is usually titrated up from a starting dose of 10 mg twice daily.

Nitrates are available as different salts and are formulated into different dosage forms. Glyceryl trinitrate (GTN) is frequently used as a sublingual spray (also as sublingual tablets). This formulation is used when the patient feels their angina symptoms commence and is used to provide acute relief. GTN is also available as a patch formulation. Isosorbide mono- and dinitrate are taken as tablets on a regular basis; they are used to prevent angina attacks. The timing of dosing of nitrates is important to prevent tolerance to their effects. Isosorbide dinitrate is available as a solution for injection for more severe cases of the condition and for facilitating angioplasty.

Ranolazine is dosed orally and is usually an add-on therapy for treating symptoms when the first-line treatment is inadequate or cannot be optimised (first-line treatments are usually beta-blockers and or calcium channel blockers).

What are the notable adverse effects to look out for?

Beta-blockers have numerous adverse effects, including bradycardia, bronchospasm, cold extremities, dizziness, and hypotension.

Calcium channel blockers. Nausea, abdominal discomfort, ankle swelling, palpitations, flushing, headache, dizziness, and hypotension.

Ivabradine. Blurred vision, bradycardia, dizziness, headache, and visual disturbances.

Nicorandil. Headache, dizziness, palpitations, flushing, nausea and vomiting, weakness, and ulceration.

Nitrates. Postural hypotension and light headedness, headache, and flushing.

Ranolazine. Asthenia, constipation, headache, dizziness, and nausea and vomiting.

What needs to be monitored?

Monitoring of cardiovascular parameters and angina symptoms is paramount for the condition. Heart rate is a factor to be considered in the administration and prescribing of ivabradine.

What drug interactions are important?

Beta-blockers interact with beta-agonists such as salbutamol. They also interact with digoxin and other drugs that affect blood pressure. Beta-blockers can mask the symptoms of hypoglycaemia.

Calcium channel blockers interact with a range of drugs such as anti-arrhythmics, anti-convulsants, ivabradine (lowering of heart rate), macrolide antibiotics and the statins, as well as grapefruit and grapefruit juice.

Ivabradine is affected by drugs that are CYP3A4 inhibitors and the starting dose needs to be adjusted to reflect this. If a medication is a CYP3A4 inhibitor concomitant use of this is often a contraindication to the use of ivabradine.

Nicorandil and the nitrates interact with phosphodiesterase inhibitors such as sildenafil. Nicorandil also interacts with non-steroidal anti-inflammatory drugs.

Ranolazine is affected by other drugs that are CYP3A4 inhibitors and inducers, statins, and drugs that prolong the QT interval.

Other considerations

Abrupt withdrawal of beta-blockers is associated with an exacerbation of angina. If beta-blockers need to be discontinued the withdrawal should be gradual.

Calcium channel blockers are often formulated in a slow or modified release form. Many of these formulations are not interchangeable and have differing bioavailability profiles.

43 Calcium Channel Blockers

These are sometimes less correctly called calcium antagonists or calcium channel antagonists.

Commonly used examples
Dihydropyridine type. Amlodipine, felodipine, lacidipine, lercanidipine, nicardipine, nifedipine
Non-dihydropyridine type. diltiazem, verapamil.

Are these drugs all the same?
Calcium channel blockers are typically considered as dihydropyridine type or non-dihydropyridine type.

What are these drugs used to treat?
Dihydropyridine type. Hypertension, angina prophylaxis.
Diltiazem. Hypertension, angina.
Verapamil. Hypertension, angina, cardiac arrhythmias.
Nimodipine. Treatment or prevention of ischaemic consequences of subarachnoid haemorrhage.

What do these drugs do?
The contraction of muscle tissue is in part mediated though the action of intracellular calcium ions. Calcium ions can enter muscle cells through the opening of specific pores in the cell membrane (termed calcium channels) in response to a depolarising action potential. Blockade of these channels prevents the movement of calcium ions into the cell in response to stimulation, reducing muscle contraction. In blood vessels, this results in vasodilatation and in the heart a reduction in inotropic, dromatropic, and chronotropic effects. As blood pressure is partly maintained through a combination of peripheral resistance and cardiac output, reducing these through vasodilatation or negative inotropic or chronotropic effects results in a reduction in blood pressure. A reduced inotropic effect and coronary vessel vasodilatation is also useful in the treatment of angina.

What's the difference between the dihydropyridines, diltiazem, and verapamil?
All of the calcium channel blockers that are used therapeutically bind to and block voltage gated, L-type calcium channels. However, the different types of calcium channel blocker have different selectivity for calcium channels in different parts of the body. The dihydropyridine type have greater selectivity for calcium channels in blood vessels and other smooth

Rapid Medicines Management for Healthcare Professionals, First Edition. Paul Deslandes, Simon Young and Ben Pitcher.
© 2020 John Wiley & Sons Ltd. Published 2020 by John Wiley & Sons Ltd.

muscle, whereas verapamil has greater selectivity for calcium channels in the heart. Diltiazem has some affinity for channels in both the heart and blood vessels.

How are these drugs given?

Regularly (usually daily or twice a day, but may be more frequently depending on the medicine and formulation) by mouth on a long-term basis for hypertension or angina.

Nimodipine is given regularly by mouth or intravenous infusion for a maximum of 21 days for the treatment or prevention of ischaemic consequences of subarachnoid haemorrhage.

Dosing

As with many medicines, initiate at a low dose and gradually titrate upwards.

Longer acting agents (e.g. amlodipine, felodipine, lacidipine) which can be given once a day are generally preferred.

There may be differences between diltiazem formulations. Patients should be maintained on the same brand to minimise variation in effect.

What are the notable adverse effects to look out for?

Ankle swelling (more common in women and the elderly and with dihydropyridines), atrioventricular block (diltiazem and verapamil), bradycardia and heart block (diltiazem and verapamil), constipation (verapamil), dizziness, dyspnoea (diltiazem), erythema (diltiazem), fatigue, flushing, gingival hyperplasia, headache, hypotension, nausea, palpitations, tachycardia, worsening of heart failure (especially diltiazem and verapamil, but all calcium channel blockers should generally be avoided).

How can the adverse effects be minimised?

Start at a low dose and use the lowest effective dose (many of the adverse effects are dose related).

Switch to an alternative type of agent (the incidence of adverse effects with dihydropyridines and non-dihydropyridines varies).

Diuretics are *not* effective in the management of ankle swelling or peripheral oedema associated with calcium channel blockers.

What needs to be monitored?

Blood pressure should be monitored in patients with hypertension.

What drug interactions are important?

Verapamil should be avoided (and diltiazem used with caution) in patients prescribed beta-blockers due to the risk of bradycardia and heart failure.

Medicines known to reduce blood pressure (e.g. alpha-blockers and other antihypertensives, tricyclic antidepressants, certain antipsychotics) may increase the risk of postural hypotension. Medicines known to increase blood pressure (e.g. non-steroidal anti-inflammatory drugs) may inhibit the antihypertensive effect of calcium channel blockers.

The maximum daily dose of simvastatin should be reduced to 20 mg in patients taking amlodipine, diltiazem or verapamil. Plasma levels of other statins may also be increased.

Diltiazem and verapamil are inhibitors of cytochrome P450 3A4. Plasma levels of medicines metabolised by this enzyme (e.g. carbamazepine) may be increased.

Verapamil is a p-glycoprotein inhibitor and may increase the plasma levels of medicines which are substrates for this transporter (e.g. digoxin).

Several of the dihydropyridines (e.g. felodipine, lercanidipine, nifedipine) as well as diltiazem and verapamil are metabolised by CYP3A4. Their effects may be increased by CYP3A4 inhibitors (e.g. azole antifungals, macrolide antibiotics, protease inhibitors) or reduced by CYP3A4 inducers (e.g. carbamazepine, phenobarbital, rifampicin, St John's wort).

Grapefruit juice has been shown to increase the bioavailability and clinical effect of felodipine. The bioavailability of other calcium channel blockers may also be increased, although the effect on blood pressure may be less significant than that seen with felodipine.

Discontinuing treatment

Abrupt discontinuation of calcium channel blockers may be associated with a withdrawal syndrome and there is some evidence to suggest an increased risk of acute myocardial infarction following withdrawal. Caution is advised.

44 Drugs for Hyperlipidaemia

Many groups of drugs are used to treat abnormal blood lipid profiles associated with different types of medically classified hyperlipidaemia (raised lipid levels). The most commonly encountered family is the statins. The statins are widely prescribed and can even be purchased over the counter.

Commonly used examples

Statins, e.g. simvastatin and atorvastatin.
Bile acid sequestrants (BASs), e.g. colestyramine.
Fibrates, e.g. bezafibrate.
Cholesterol absorption inhibitors, e.g. ezetimibe.
Nicotinic acid derivatives, e.g. acipimox and nicotinic acid.
PCSK9 inhibitors, e.g. alirocumab and evolcumab.

Are these drugs all the same?

Whilst all of these drugs are used to treat hyperlipidaemia, they are grouped according to their mechanism of action, which varies significantly. The PCSK9 inhibitors are examples of biologic medicines and unlike the other drugs listed are large complex molecules given by injection.

What are these drugs used to treat?

These drugs all help to reduce levels of lipids in the body. Lipid-lowering agents are used to treat hyperlipidaemia and to prevent the consequences of hyperlipidaemia, e.g. cardiovascular disease. They are used for both primary and secondary prevention of cardiovascular disease. Many lipid-lowering agents are used to treat specific subtypes of hyperlipidaemia, e.g. hypercholesterolemia, hypertriglyceridemia, and genetic/familial hypercholesterolemia.

Statins are indicated in treating a range of abnormal lipid profiles, including primary hypercholesterolemia, heterozygous familial hypercholesterolemia, and primary and secondary prevention of cardiovascular disease. The statins' pharmacodynamic action suggests they are effective in lowering low-density lipoprotein (LDL) cholesterol but less effective at lowering triglyceride levels. Fibrates, on the other hand, are more effective at lowering triglycerides than the statins. The medications used will depend very much on the nature of the patient's dyslipidaemia. PCSK9 inhibitors are typically only used in patients who have not responded well to other therapies.

Rapid Medicines Management for Healthcare Professionals, First Edition. Paul Deslandes, Simon Young and Ben Pitcher.
© 2020 John Wiley & Sons Ltd. Published 2020 by John Wiley & Sons Ltd.

What's the difference between different types?

Statins lower LDL cholesterol by inhibiting an enzyme (HMGCoA reductase) that is involved in the endogenous synthesis of cholesterol.

BASs increase the elimination of bile acids from the body and the body utilises cholesterol from the blood to produce new bile acids (thus 'dragging' cholesterol from the blood). Fibrates have a wide range of actions that reduce LDL, very low-density lipoprotein (VLDL), and triglycerides.

Ezetimibe reduces the absorption of cholesterol from the gastrointestinal tract.

The nicotinic acid derivatives prevent the release of fatty acids from adipose tissue and decrease the concentration of VLDL and LDL in the blood. This results in lowering of triglyceride and cholesterol levels.

PCSK9 inhibitors are monoclonal antibodies that bind to, and render inactive, a specific protein that results in an increased rate of LDL cholesterol uptake into the liver.

How are these drugs given?

There is a wide range of lipid-lowering agents; they are usually dosed orally. The statins are usually presented as capsule, oral liquid or tablet forms. The BASs are oral tablets or granules, and the fibrates are tablets or modified release tablets. Ezetimibe is a tablet and nicotinic acid is available as a capsule. There are compound formulations available that combine two or more families, e.g. Inegy®, which combines simvastatin 20, 40, or 80mg with ezetimibe 10mg in one tablet. Another example is Cholib® (a combination of fenofibrate 145mg with either 20 or 40mg of simvastatin).

Dosing

Statins are dosed according to their indication. Starting doses are often titrated up to the indicated dose to maximise adherence. BASs are often initiated at a staring dose and the dose raised to achieve target lipid levels. The fibrates are dosed in a similar way to the statins and BASs. Ezetimibe is given at a fixed dose of 10mg daily in adults and children over 10years of age. Nicotinic acid is dosed orally at two dose tiers (150 or 300mg daily).

What are the notable adverse effects to look out for?

Statins are commonly associated with muscle pain. More serious muscle-related problems, such as myopathy, myositis, and rhabdomyolysis, are rare. Monitoring creatinine kinase is key if problematic symptoms are present in the patient. Other broader adverse effects, such as abnormal liver function tests, headache, fatigue, and gastrointestinal disturbance, are noted in the literature. The BASs have gastrointestinal side effects and bleeding disorders associated with their use. The fibrates, ezetimibe, and nicotinic acid (and derivatives) have associated gastrointestinal side effects, fatigue, muscle related adverse effects, and headaches.

How can the adverse effects be minimised?

Monitoring of factors such as liver function and creatinine kinase prior to statin treatment may help to avoid initiation in patients at increased risk of adverse effects, such as those with impaired liver function and those with unexplained muscle pain. Drug interactions may increase the risk of adverse effects, and concomitant use of interacting drugs may require dosage alterations (see below).

What needs to be monitored?

As well as monitoring the patient's lipid profile to ensure the drug is efficacious, statin therapy requires monitoring of liver function tests before treatment and repeats of those tests within 3 and 12 months of commencement of the drug. This monitoring may be more frequent if there are signs/symptoms associated with hepatotoxicity. Serum transaminases are a key marker. Creatinine kinase is sometimes measured, especially if patients are experiencing muscle pain (see the section on adverse effects).

What drug interactions are important?

Some drug interactions occur between statins and other drugs that increase the incidence of myopathy associated with statin use. Statin levels are increased by macrolide antibacterials such as erythromycin, the imidazole antifungals, certain antiviral drugs, ciclosporin, and calcium channel blockers. These interactions can result in an increased risk of adverse effects and often necessitate dosage alterations of the statin (refer to the *British National Formulary* for further information). Concurrent use of statins and fibrates can result in an increased risk of myopathy. Some statins also interact with grapefruit juice (drug–food interaction).

The BASs interact with the coumarins and phenindione in a potentially hazardous manner. Ezetimibe interacts with rosuvastatin in a hazardous manner and also with the immunosuppressant ciclosporin. The fibrates interact with a range of drugs, including colchicine, coumarins, phenindione, and the statins.

Other considerations

Lomitapide is one of the newer lipid-lowering agents. It is used under specialist supervision. The drug is currently a black triangle drug (▼) and has very specific indications. This means it will be encountered less frequently in clinical practice than the statins. Simvastatin 10 mg is available to the public over the counter from pharmacies for certain indications.

45 Antihistamines

Commonly used examples

Sedating. Alimemazine, chlorphenamine, cinnarizine, diphenhydramine, hydroxyzine, promethazine.

Non-sedating. Acrivastine, cetirizine, desloratadine, fexofenadine, levocetirizine, loratadine.

Are these drugs all the same?

Antihistamines can be divided into those that antagonise (block) the histamine H_1 receptor (and are the focus of this chapter) and those that inhibit the histamine H_2 receptor and influence gastric acid secretion (see Chapter 34).

The histamine H_1 receptor antagonists considered in this chapter are usually divided into two groups: the older sedating drugs and the more recently developed non-sedating drugs.

What are these drugs used to treat?

Histamine H_1 antagonists help to relieve symptoms of allergy (e.g. allergic rhinitis, hayfever, drug allergy, food allergy), as well as atopic dermatitis, pruritus, and urticaria.

Sedating antihistamines are available to purchase over the counter from pharmacies for the treatment of temporary, mild insomnia.

What do these drugs do?

Histamine is a chemical messenger with a number of different functions in the body. It forms part of the immune system response to allergens, being released from mast cells following degranulation and acting on histamine H_1 receptors. This results in symptoms of allergy such as redness, itching, and swelling. Histamine is also associated with the release of acid from the parietal cells lining the stomach, an effect that is mediated through histamine H_2 receptors.

Antihistamines inhibit the effect of histamine at its receptors. Antihistamines used in the treatment of allergy reduce activity at the histamine H_1 receptor and are the focus of this chapter. Antihistamines acting at histamine H_2 receptors inhibit acid secretion and are sometimes used to treat gastro-oesophageal reflux disease and peptic ulcer, described in Chapter 34.

What's the difference between sedating and non-sedating antihistamines?

Both sedating and non-sedating antihistamines inhibit the effect of histamine at the histamine H_1 receptor. This helps to reduce symptoms of allergy.

Rapid Medicines Management for Healthcare Professionals, First Edition. Paul Deslandes, Simon Young and Ben Pitcher.
© 2020 John Wiley & Sons Ltd. Published 2020 by John Wiley & Sons Ltd.

Sedating antihistamines are able to cross the blood–brain barrier. The resulting action in the central nervous system leads to a sedating effect. Several of the sedating antihistamines also have antimuscarinic properties and this may be associated with adverse drug reactions such as constipation, dry mouth urinary retention, and confusion (particularly in the elderly).

Non-sedating antihistamines have been developed more recently and are less able to cross the blood–brain barrier. This results in less sedation, although the anti-allergy effect is maintained. The newer antihistamines have fewer antimuscarinic effects and are therefore less likely to be associated with adverse effects such as dry mouth, constipation, and urinary retention. The newer non-sedating antihistamines desloratadine and levocetirizine are related to loratadine and cetirizine, respectively. Desloratadine is an active metabolite of the drug loratadine, whilst levocetirizine is one of the enantiomers (chemicals with mirror-image structures) of cetirizine.

How are these drugs given?

Regularly or as required (usually daily or twice a day, but may be more frequently depending upon the medicine) by mouth, on a short-term basis to treat allergic reactions. If used for insomnia, a single dose is taken at night and should only be used on a short-term basis for temporary, mild insomnia.

As a single dose, by intravenous or intramuscular injection for emergency treatment of anaphylaxis.

Dosing

Antihistamines are typically initiated at treatment doses. The newer, non-sedating agents (e.g. cetirizine) can be dosed once a day, whilst some of the older sedating medicines (e.g. chlorphenamine) are shorter acting and are therefore dosed more frequently.

What are the notable adverse effects to look out for?

Antihistamines are generally well tolerated although drowsiness can be notable in sedating antihistamines, but less common in non-sedating antihistamines. Sedation can continue the day after taking sedating drugs, resulting in a 'hangover' effect. There are reports of sedating drugs being misused and taken in increasing doses on a long-term basis.

In addition to sedation, the older agents may rarely cause paradoxical excitation. They should not be given to children in over-the-counter cough and cold remedies. Some of the older agents have antimuscarinic effects (e.g. diphenhydramine) and may therefore cause blurred vision, constipation, and urinary retention. Hydroxyzine is associated with a small increase in the risk of cardiac QT interval prolongation. QT interval prolongation may be associated with an increased risk of cardiac arrhythmia.

How can the adverse effects be minimised?

As with many medicines the lowest effective dose should be used for the shortest possible duration. Selecting a non-sedating antihistamine or one without antimuscarinic effects will help to avoid these adverse drug reactions.

Hydroxyzine should be avoided in patients with other risk factors for QT interval prolongation and in patients taking other drugs known to prolong the QT interval.

What drug interactions are important?

An additive effect may be seen with other sedating medicines (e.g. benzodiazepines, barbiturates, tricyclic antidepressants, alcohol), even with the non-sedating antihistamines. Similarly, the use of antimuscarinic medicines in combination with those antihistamines with antimuscarinic properties may lead to additive adverse effects. This is a particular concern in the elderly, where the combined use of antimuscarinic medicines (sometimes termed anticholinergic burden) can cause confusion.

Hydroxyzine – Other medicines with the potential to prolong the QT interval (e.g. anti-arrhythmics, tricyclic antidepressants, methadone) or to affect electrolyte (in particular potassium) levels, which may increase the risk of cardiac arrhythmias.

Discontinuing treatment

Following short-term use, antihistamines can typically be discontinued without particular concern. However, if there is evidence of misuse of high doses over a long period, a gradual dose reduction may be required.

46 Bronchodilators

Bronchodilators are used to increase the diameter of the bronchioles and therefore allow an easier passage of air into and out of the lungs. They do this by different mechanisms and have different durations of action.

Commonly used examples

Adrenoceptor agonists. Salbutamol (e.g. Ventolin®), salmeterol (e.g. Serevent®), formoterol.
Muscarinic antagonists. Ipratropium (e.g. Atrovent®), tiotropium.
Xanthines. Theophylline, aminophylline.

Are these drugs all the same?

The bronchodilators above can be divided into three groups according to their different mechanisms of action. The adrenoceptor agonists and muscarinic antagonists are typically given via inhalation, whereas xanthines are more commonly given orally or by injection.

What are these drugs used to treat?

Bronchodilators are used to improve the passage of air into the lungs. This is usually to counteract a narrowing of the small airways brought about by airway inflammation or spasm of the bronchiolar smooth muscle. They can be used in many types of respiratory disease, but are most commonly seen in patients with asthma, chronic obstructive pulmonary disease (COPD) or respiratory tract infection.

What do these drugs do?

The bronchiole walls contain a layer of smooth muscle. This smooth muscle can be contracted or allowed to relax in order to allow the bronchiole to either constrict or dilate. This is normally controlled by the autonomic nervous system. The parasympathetic nervous system stimulates muscarinic receptors on the muscle, causing it to constrict. The sympathetic nervous system stimulates adrenoceptors, causing the muscle to relax and the bronchiole to dilate.

The majority of bronchodilators either block the action of the parasympathetic nervous system or stimulate the sympathetic nervous system. However, the xanthines act on the smooth muscle and facilitate its relaxation.

When considering the treatment of respiratory diseases such as asthma medicines are often categorised as *relievers* or *preventers*. Relievers (such as salbutamol) have fast onset of action and shorter duration of action; they may be administered in response to a respiratory decline (such as an asthma attack). This is in contrast to preventers (typically inhaled

Rapid Medicines Management for Healthcare Professionals, First Edition. Paul Deslandes, Simon Young and Ben Pitcher.
© 2020 John Wiley & Sons Ltd. Published 2020 by John Wiley & Sons Ltd.

steroids), which have a longer duration of action and a slower onset of action; these are intended to prevent attacks from occurring in the first place.

What's the difference between different types?

Adrenoceptor agonists stimulate the receptors which would typically be stimulated by adrenaline or noradrenaline. There are different subsets of adrenoceptors which are found on different organs of the body. The beta-2 adrenergic receptor is found in the airways and triggers bronchodilation in the presence of an agonist. The adrenoceptor agonists used in respiratory disorders are often referred to as *beta-2 agonists*.

Antimuscarinic bronchodilators work by preventing bronchoconstriction initiated by the parasympathetic nervous system. The parasympathetic nervous system would normally trigger bronchoconstriction by releasing acetylcholine onto a subtype of receptors called muscarinic receptors. Blocking these receptors with muscarinic antagonists blocks the parasympathetic stimulation and therefore lessens the bronchoconstriction and increases airway diameter.

Theophylline and aminophylline act directly on the smooth muscle and trigger bronchodilation.

Bronchodilators can also be divided into groups based upon their duration of action often termed short-acting beta agonists (SABAs), long-acting beta agonists (LABAs), or long-acting muscarinic antagonists (LAMAs). SABAs (such as salbutamol) have a fast onset of action but short duration of action and are used as relievers.

LABAs and LAMAs have a longer duration of action and are used as maintenance therapy to help keep the airways open throughout the day; they are not *preventers* and do not replace the need for a preventer. Most have a slow onset of action, which would make them dangerously ineffective in the treatment of acute symptoms and therefore they cannot be used as a reliever. However, there are some exceptions to this; some LABAs, such as formoterol, have a long duration of action (making it a LABA) but also have a fast onset of action, making it effective as a reliever and a maintenance therapy.

How are these drugs given?

The most commonly used bronchodilators are inhaled using some form of metered dose inhaler (MDI) device or via a nebuliser. However, some adrenoceptor agonists can be given orally (e.g. salbutamol syrup) or in emergency situations, subcutaneously or intravenously (e.g. salbutamol or terbutaline). Bronchodilators are often combined with other respiratory drugs (such as inhaled corticosteroids) in a single inhaler device to improve patient adherence particularly in relation to preventer therapy.

There is a huge range of inhaler devices available across the different varieties and brands of bronchodilator. The differences between these devices and issues associated with their use are discussed in greater depth in Chapter 17. Poor administration technique is a common problem, and inhaler technique should be checked to ensure that patients are using their device correctly.

Theophylline is given orally and aminophylline intravenously to relieve acute exacerbations. These drugs have narrow therapeutic ranges (the difference between a therapeutic and toxic dose is small), therefore care is required.

Dosing

Dosing of bronchodilators via MDIs is usually measured by the number of actuations or 'puffs' as each actuation should provide a consistent metered dose. Relievers are typically prescribed to be used as required to relieve symptoms and can be given in high doses (up to 15 puffs every 10 minutes) if necessary.

Theophylline is dosed orally twice per day. It is formulated as modified release tablets or capsules. The different products may release the drug slightly differently and are therefore not interchangeable. These drugs have narrow therapeutic ranges (the difference between a therapeutic and toxic dose is small); therapeutic drug monitoring is required.

What are the notable adverse effects to look out for?

Adverse effects of bronchodilators vary depending on the specific pharmacology of the drug. Adrenoceptor agonists mimic the effects of adrenaline or noradrenaline and tend to cause adverse effects such as tachycardia and tremor.

Antimuscarinic drugs block the action of the parasympathetic nervous system, therefore the side effects of these drugs include drying of secretions (particularly dry mouth) and gastrointestinal disturbance.

Theophylline (and aminophylline) can cause side effects such as gastric disturbance, headache, and arrhythmias. Toxicity can occur if plasma levels get too high, causing convulsions and dangerous arrhythmias.

How can the adverse effects be minimised?

Adverse effects of bronchodilators are not easily avoided and may have to be endured if they are due to the need for high dosing in emergency situations. Administration locally via inhalation helps to reduce the dose and associated adverse effects compared to systemic dosing. The risk of adverse effects (and toxicity) of theophylline can be reduced by careful dosing and therapeutic drug monitoring.

What needs to be monitored?

Bronchodilators are usually given in response to respiratory illness. If patients are requiring additional bronchodilators in an acute setting then it is important to monitor the patient's oxygen status and respiratory rate to ensure that the status is improving and not deteriorating.

Patients with chronic respiratory disease may have regular peak flow tests. These can be a good measure of airway obstruction and predictor of further deterioration.

The risk of theophylline toxicity can be reduced by monitoring of plasma levels, taken after commencing the drug or after any changes in dosing regimen.

What drug interactions are important?

Theophylline has the capacity to interact with a number of medications, particularly antimicrobials and cardiac medication. This can be problematic due to its narrow therapeutic range.

47 Oxygen

Commonly used examples of oxygen delivery
Oxygen mask
Nasal cannula (specs)

Are these drugs all the same?
By definition, all oxygen therapy delivers the same drug, oxygen. However, there are distinct differences in how the oxygen is supplied and delivered.

What are these drugs used to treat?
Oxygen therapy is used in circumstances where there is insufficient oxygen in the blood (hypoxaemia) and therefore insufficient oxygen available to the tissues to undertake aerobic respiration. This is typically due to some form of disease of the respiratory system, which is either preventing the appropriate flow of air (and the oxygen within) from adequately reaching the lungs or where a problem with the alveolar tissue means that gaseous exchange is impeded. There are also circumstances where an issue with the blood itself prevents or reduces its ability to carry oxygen, or where the flow of blood to a given tissue is reduced. In these situations, increasing the amount of available oxygen can facilitate oxygen delivery to tissues and organs.

What do these drugs do?
Oxygen is a normal constituent of air and is essential for normal cellular respiration. Whilst it is a natural part of the air that we breathe, when we administer it to patients we consider it to be a drug and therefore follow the same principles as with any other medication.

How are these drugs given?
Hospital medical oxygen
Within a hospital environment, oxygen is typically delivered to the bedside via a network of pipes. Specialised taps are attached to access ports which can be found at the head of the bed. Some clinical areas have both oxygen and 'air' ports. Medical air may be used with nebulisers when increased oxygen is not indicated or is potentially harmful (such as in patients with type 2 respiratory depression). It is therefore important to check that any oxygen delivery equipment is attached to the correct port.

Rapid Medicines Management for Healthcare Professionals, First Edition. Paul Deslandes, Simon Young and Ben Pitcher.
© 2020 John Wiley & Sons Ltd. Published 2020 by John Wiley & Sons Ltd.

Oxygen cylinders

Oxygen cylinders provide a certain degree of portability, allowing the patient to receive oxygen whilst away from the bed area or even out and about in the community. However, these metal containers filled with compressed oxygen can be quite heavy and have a finite quantity of oxygen, which means that they can run out. Before use, the capacity and content of a cylinder should be assessed and consideration should be made about whether there is enough oxygen to adequately supply the patient.

Concentrators

Oxygen concentrators use an electric motor to compress and concentrate room air into a supply of nearly pure oxygen (the concentrator's output is typically around 95% oxygen mixed with other atmospheric gasses). These are more commonly used for patients who require oxygen therapy at home.

Delivery devices

Whatever the source of the oxygen it can be delivered through a variety of devices.

Nasal cannula (often referred to as nasal specs) is a set of plastic tubing looped behind the ears and running across the front of the face, sitting just under the nose. In the centre of the loop are two tubes, which, when the oxygen is passed through the tube, allow oxygen to be pumped directly into the nose. Nasal cannula are a convenient way of increasing the inspired oxygen of a patient without obstructing their mouth and thereby not impeding eating or talking. However, they are only capable of supplying small amounts of additional oxygen (often described as low flow) and therefore cannot be used with patients who require significant oxygen support.

Oxygen masks are widely used as a means of delivering oxygen to patients. There are a huge variety of different masks which can deliver an equally large variety of oxygen concentrations. It is important to ensure you have fully read the instructions for the type of mask you are using in order to ensure that the patient receives the maximum benefit.

In more serious circumstances oxygen can also be delivered via a tube inserted down the trachea and held in place by an inflatable cuff, these are termed endotracheal tubes (ETTs). ETTs are usually only used in emergency situations, when a patient is undergoing surgery or in critical care where they are used in conjunction with ventilators. ETTs cannot be tolerated by a conscious patient and are not a long-term solution. Should this level of support be required for extended periods, a tracheostomy tube may be inserted through an opening which has been cut through the skin directly into the trachea. Tracheostomy tubes are used in critical care to allow long-term use of ventilatory support, or where disease or damage means that it must be used as an alternative air entry point for normal breathing.

Dosing

The dosing of oxygen therapy can be discussed in two distinct ways. The first method relates to the flow rate of oxygen (measured in litres per minute) being delivered through the equipment (e.g. 'nasal specs on 2 litres'). This method is practical and objective, as it describes the equipment to be used and the flow rate to be set. However, it is important to remember that different delivery devices on the same flow rate can provide radically different amounts of oxygen to the patient.

The alternative method relates to what (as a result of the additional oxygen supplied) is the actual percentage of oxygen in the air that the patient is breathing. This is described as the fraction of inspired oxygen (FiO_2). Normal room air is 21% oxygen, a patient using 'nasal specs on 2 litres' will have an inspired oxygen of around 30%. However, this can sometimes be inexact as the amount of oxygen actually inspired may vary depending on factors such as the respiratory rate and even if the patient has their mouth open or closed.

What are the notable adverse effects to look out for?

Medical oxygen has no humidity (there is no water vapour in it). This can cause it to dry the patient's mouth, airway, and even lungs.

Where nasal specs or masks are held in place for extended periods of time, they can rub and cause damage where they are in contact with the skin. This is particularly noticeable behind the ears and on the nose.

How can the adverse effects be minimised?

Use of humidification can help to ensure that there is adequate water vapour in the oxygen supply. This is essentially a bottle of water through which the air is bubbled before being delivered to the patient.

Patients receiving oxygen therapy should also receive adequate oral care to ensure that the drying effects of the oxygen are not causing problems. It is possible to use some form of lubricant to help keep the lips protected and prevent the rubbing of the mask or nasal specs. However, there is a potential fire risk from using a petroleum (or other oil-based) lubricant with oxygen.

What needs to be monitored?

Respiratory rate and oxygen saturations should be monitored closely to ensure that the oxygen provision is adequate for the patient's needs. A 3% drop in oxygen saturations below the target range for a patient should be reported and the patient reviewed. Patients with chronic respiratory problems who receive oxygen therapy on an ongoing basis may not need to be monitored so closely.

Blood gasses may be undertaken for acutely unwell patients. This will allow a more accurate measure of the oxygen and carbon dioxide levels in the blood, as well as the blood pH.

Other considerations

Smoking is one of the more common causes of respiratory disease that may result in the use of oxygen therapy. It is possible that even though smoking may have caused the disease, a patient may continue to smoke and even attempt to continue smoking whilst receiving oxygen therapy. This presents a significant risk, as the oxygen is a significant aid to combustion. The potential for the patient setting themselves alight is real and could be fatal.

Type 2 respiratory failure is a form of chronic respiratory disease in which patients become desensitised to carbon dioxide levels. It is therefore possible that if they receive too much oxygen their respiratory rate can drop and they can become hypercapnic. Because of this, patients with this form of respiratory failure are often given a lower dose of oxygen therapy than might be expected.

Oxygen is a drug and therefore should be treated as such. However, if a patient is clearly in respiratory distress it is reasonable to commence them on oxygen whilst you seek help or review from more a senior colleague.

48 Antipsychotics

Antipsychotics are sometimes (rarely) called 'neuroleptics' or 'major tranquilisers'.

Commonly used examples

Typical. Chlorpromazine, haloperidol, flupentixol, sulpiride, zuclopenthixol.

Atypical. Amisulpride, aripiprazole, lurasidone, olanzapine, paliperidone, quetiapine, risperidone, clozapine (see Chapter 49).

Are these drugs all the same?

Antipsychotics are usually divided into two groups: 'typical' and 'atypical', sometimes called 'first' and 'second' generation antipsychotics, respectively.

What are these drugs used to treat?

Typical

Commonly. Schizophrenia, other psychotic illness, bipolar mania/hypomania, acute agitation.

Less commonly. Nausea and vomiting, intractable hiccup, Tourette's syndrome.

Atypical

Commonly. Schizophrenia, other psychotic illness, bipolar mania, maintenance treatment of bipolar affective disorder, acute agitation and disturbed behaviour in schizophrenia or mania.

Less commonly. Bipolar depression, adjunctive treatment of major depression, behavioural and psychiatric symptoms of dementia (short term only), aggression in conduct disorder (short term only).

What do these drugs do?

Symptoms of psychosis are believed to be associated with changes in the activity of dopaminergic neurons in certain brain regions. The therapeutic effect and some adverse effects of antipsychotics are thought to be mediated through blockade of the dopamine D_2 receptor. Blockade of other neurotransmitter receptors (e.g. muscarinic, serotonergic, alpha-adrenergic) contributes to adverse effects.

Rapid Medicines Management for Healthcare Professionals, First Edition. Paul Deslandes, Simon Young and Ben Pitcher.
© 2020 John Wiley & Sons Ltd. Published 2020 by John Wiley & Sons Ltd.

What's the difference between typical and atypical antipsychotics?

Typical antipsychotics have been available since the 1950s and are potent blockers of the dopamine D_2 receptor (in addition to many other receptors). As a result, they are typically associated with a group of neurological side effects, termed extra-pyramidal side effects (EPSEs) as well as elevation of prolactin levels. Effects at other receptors and ion channels lead to adverse effects such as postural hypotension, sedation, and cardiac conduction abnormalities.

Atypical antipsychotics have been available since the 1990s, and also block the dopamine D_2 receptor. However, they generally have a lower affinity for this receptor than typical antipsychotics and have a greater affinity for the serotonin 5-HT_{2A} receptor. It appears that this leads to a reduced incidence of EPSEs. Because each individual atypical antipsychotic can inhibit the effects of a variety of other neurotransmitters and receptors, there is a varied side effect profile across the group. This can include weight gain, metabolic syndrome, increased prolactin levels, and sedation.

How are these drugs given?

Regularly (usually daily or twice a day, but may be more frequently depending upon the medicine), by mouth, on a long-term basis to treat chronic mental illness.

Regularly (between weekly and monthly or three monthly), as a long-acting intramuscular injection on a long-term basis to treat chronic mental illness.

As required, by mouth or short-acting intramuscular injection on a short-term basis to treat acute behavioural disturbance associated with mental illness.

Regularly or as required, by mouth or intramuscular injection to treat nausea and vomiting.

Dosing

As with many medicines, initiate at a low dose and gradually titrate upwards. This is important to help minimise postural hypotension and sedation early in treatment. Patients with first episode illness will generally respond to lower doses than those with more chronic illness who are not treatment naïve. Patients who are previously antipsychotic naïve, the elderly, young women, and patients with bipolar affective disorder may all be more sensitive to the adverse effects of antipsychotics and particular caution is needed in these groups.

What are the notable adverse effects to look out for?

Typical. EPSE, prolactin elevation, sedation, postural hypotension, QT interval prolongation (especially haloperidol and pimozide), sexual dysfunction, constipation, blurred vision, dry mouth.

Atypical. Weight gain and metabolic syndrome (more common with olanzapine and quetiapine), sedation, prolactin elevation (more common with risperidone), postural hypotension, QT interval prolongation (more common with quetiapine and amisulpride), sexual dysfunction.

How can the adverse effects be minimised?

General. The dose may be cautiously reduced to the lowest effective for the patient or the antipsychotic switched to an alternative with a different side effect profile.

EPSE. Pseudoparkinsonism – anticholinergic medicines (e.g. procyclidine) can be used or switch to an atypical agent. Tardive dyskinesia – the antipsychotic may be switched to an atypical agent (this may worsen symptoms in the short term). Akathisia – generally difficult to treat and may require switching to an atypical agent. Acute dystonia – anticholinergic medicines (e.g. procyclidine) may be used (given intramuscularly if symptoms are severe) or the antipsychotic switched to an atypical agent.

What needs to be monitored?

This will depend upon the specific medicine, but commonly as follows:

Typical. Electrocardiogram (ECG) at baseline and following dose change, then annually. Serum prolactin, weight, blood glucose.
Atypical. ECG at baseline and following dose changes, then annually (amisulpride), weight, blood glucose (or HbA1C), plasma lipids at baseline, frequently for the first year, then annually (olanzapine, quetiapine), serum prolactin (risperidone, paliperidone).

What drug interactions are important?

Use of other medicines with the potential to prolong the QT interval (e.g. anti-arrhythmics, tricyclic antidepressants, methadone) or affect electrolyte (potassium) levels may increase the risk of cardiac arrythmias. Use of other sedating medicines (e.g. benzodiazepines, barbiturates, tricyclic antidepressants, alcohol) may increase the risk of drowsiness. Use of medicines causing hypotension (e.g. alpha- and beta-blockers) may increase the risk of postural hypotension. Use of medicines affecting metabolic liver (cytochrome P450) enzymes (e.g. erythromycin, clarithromycin, fluoxetine, venlafaxine, itraconazole, phenytoin, carbamazepine, phenobarbital, rifampicin) may increase or decrease levels of certain antipsychotics. Use of other anticholinergic medicines can increase the anticholinergic burden and may lead to confusion and falls, particularly in elderly patients (although these medicines may be used to treat EPSEs with typical antipsychotics).

Discontinuing treatment

When discontinuing, the dose of antipsychotics should normally be reduced gradually before stopping to minimise the risk of withdrawal symptoms and recurrence of symptoms. Similarly, when switching from one antipsychotic to another, a cross-tapering approach is commonly used, where the dose of the first medicine is gradually reduced as the dose of the second medicine is gradually increased. This approach may not always be appropriate and if in doubt specialist advice should be sought.

49 Clozapine

Brand names include Clozaril®, Denzapine®, and Zaponex®.

What is clozapine?

Clozapine is an *atypical antipsychotic* that was first developed in the 1960s. Following a number of deaths associated with adverse events it was withdrawn from the market. However, it was later shown to be effective in the management of schizophrenia that had responded poorly to other antipsychotic treatments (sometimes known as treatment refractory schizophrenia) and was reintroduced. In the UK, the marketing authorisation requires careful monitoring for adverse effects (see section on monitoring).

Clozapine is a weak blocker of the dopamine D_2 receptor and also inhibits the effect of serotonin at the serotonin 5-HT_{2A} and 5-HT_{2C} receptors, as well as having effects on alpha-adrenergic and muscarinic acetylcholine receptors. It has an active metabolite (norclozapine) which is a muscarinic receptor agonist.

What is clozapine used to treat?

Refractory schizophrenia.

Psychosis associated with Parkinson's disease.

What does clozapine do?

Symptoms of psychosis are believed to be associated with changes in the functioning of dopaminergic neurons in certain brain regions. The therapeutic effect of clozapine is not fully understood, but may in part be mediated through blockade of the dopamine D_2 receptor. Effects on other neurotransmitter (e.g. glutamate) actions may also play a part, and blockade of muscarinic, serotonergic, histaminergic, and alpha-adrenergic receptors contributes to adverse effects.

How is clozapine given?

Regularly (usually twice a day or daily), by mouth, on a long-term basis to treat chronic mental illness.

Dosing

A gradual dose increase is particularly important with clozapine; it is initiated at a low dose and gradually titrated upwards. This is important to help minimise adverse effects (particularly postural hypotension and tachycardia) early in treatment. Dose titration usually begins at 12.5 mg and is increased in steps of 12.5–50 mg on a daily basis over two weeks.

Rapid Medicines Management for Healthcare Professionals, First Edition. Paul Deslandes, Simon Young and Ben Pitcher.

The initial target dose is typically 300 mg per day (usually in divided doses), with further dosage adjustments based on patient response, adverse effects, and therapeutic drug monitoring.

What are the notable adverse effects to look out for?

Side effects of clozapine may be potentially life threatening and require careful monitoring.

Changes in bone marrow function and blood cell formation may lead to neutropenia, thrombocytopenia, and agranulocytosis, which requires monitoring (see below) although this is relatively uncommon.

Constipation is a common side effect, which should be carefully monitored as it has been associated with fatal bowel obstruction.

Common side effects on initiation include postural hypotension, hypertension, tachycardia, and sedation.

Other common side effects include weight gain and metabolic syndrome, sedation, and hypersalivation. Clozapine lowers the seizure threshold in a dose-dependent manner.

How can the adverse effects be minimised?

Consider cautiously reducing the dose to the lowest effective for the patient. Note that because clozapine is used for patients who have failed to respond to other antipsychotics, switching to a different agent is unlikely to be an effective strategy for managing side effects.

Constipation may be managed with laxatives and lifestyle interventions. Weight gain may be managed with dietary and lifestyle advice. Co-prescription of other medication (e.g. metformin) may be considered in some cases. Seizure prophylaxis with sodium valproate can be used in those with high clozapine plasma levels. Hypersalivation is often difficult to manage and responds poorly to treatment. Anticholinergic medication such as hyoscine and pirenzepine (unlicensed in the UK) can be tried, but may also worsen constipation. Sedation may improve with continued treatment, but can be significant and difficult to manage. Reducing the morning clozapine dose and co-prescription of aripiprazole have been attempted.

What needs to be monitored?

Full blood count monitoring is required as part of the marketing authorisation for clozapine and the patient must be registered with the monitoring scheme of the relevant pharmaceutical company. A full blood count including white cells, neutrophils, eosinophils, and platelets is required prior to treatment, at weekly intervals for the first 18 weeks of treatment, fortnightly for the remainder of the first year, and monthly thereafter. Results are monitored using a traffic light system whereby a green result indicates that a patient can continue treatment, an amber result indicates that a patient requires closer full blood count monitoring, and a red result requires immediate discontinuation of treatment.

Other recommended monitoring: Electrocardiogram at baseline and following dose change, then annually. Weight, blood glucose (or HbA1C), plasma lipids at baseline, frequently for the first year, then annually.

Therapeutic plasma levels may be used to guide dosing requirements and provide an indication of patient adherence. The therapeutic range (trough level) is estimated to be between 350 and 500 micrograms l^{-1} whilst an increased risk of seizures has been associated with higher plasma levels.

What drug interactions are important?

Medicines which increase the risk of blood disorders, for example carbamazepine, cytotoxics, phenothiazine antipsychotics, and some antibiotics (e.g. co-trimoxazole) should be avoided. Use of other sedating medicines (e.g. benzodiazepines, barbiturates, tricyclic antidepressants) and alcohol may increase the risk of drowsiness. Medicines inhibiting metabolic liver (cytochrome P450) enzymes (e.g. erythromycin, clarithromycin, fluoxetine) may increase clozapine levels, increasing the risk of adverse effects. Medicines inducing metabolic liver (cytochrome P450) enzymes (e.g. phenytoin, phenobarbital, rifampicin) may reduce clozapine levels, reducing its effectiveness. Cigarette smoking reduces the clozapine plasma concentration. Any plans to stop smoking should be discussed with the care team, as increased levels and toxicity may occur during smoking cessation. Anticholinergic medicines and other medicines may increase the risk of constipation. Use of other medicines with the potential to prolong the QT interval (e.g. anti-arrhythmics, tricyclic antidepressants, methadone) may increase the risk of cardiac arrhythmias. Use of other medicines causing hypotension (e.g. alpha-blockers, calcium channel blockers, and angiotensin converting enzyme [ACE] inhibitors) may increase the risk of postural hypotension.

Discontinuing treatment

If a patient experiences a red blood result (see 'What needs to be monitored?' above), treatment must be stopped immediately.

Because clozapine is generally used when other antipsychotics have been ineffective, switching to another antipsychotic may be ineffective. If clozapine is discontinued, the dose should normally be reduced gradually before stopping to minimise the risk of withdrawal effects and recurrence of symptoms. Similarly, when switching from one antipsychotic to another, a cross-tapering approach is commonly used whereby the dose of the first medicine is gradually reduced as the dose of the second medicine is gradually increased. This approach may not always be appropriate and if in doubt specialist advice should be sought.

50 Antidepressants

Commonly used examples

Selective serotonin reuptake inhibitors (SSRIs). Citalopram, escitalopram, fluoxetine, fluvoxamine, paroxetine, sertraline.

Serotonin and noradrenaline reuptake inhibitors (SNRIs). Duloxetine, venlafaxine.

Tricyclic antidepressants (TCAs). Amitriptyline, clomipramine, dosulepin, doxepin, imipramine, lofepramine, nortriptyline, trimipramine.

Monoamine oxidase inhibitors (MAOIs). Isocarboxazid, moclobemide, phenelzine, tranylcypromine.

Other. Agomelatine, mianserin, mirtazapine, reboxetine, trazodone, vortioxetine.

Are these drugs all the same?

Antidepressants are usually divided into different groups according to either their mechanism of action or their chemical structure. Drugs from the same group typically have similar pharmacodynamic properties, but drugs from different groups may vary significantly.

What are these drugs used to treat?

Antidepressants are most commonly used to treat major depressive illness. However, they are also used to treat a number of other psychiatric (e.g. obsessive-compulsive disorder, generalised anxiety disorder, eating disorders) and physical disorders (e.g. pain and urinary incontinence).

What do these drugs do?

The majority of antidepressants increase levels of one or more neurotransmitter in the synaptic cleft. They achieve this through different mechanisms, including neurotransmitter reuptake inhibition, enzyme inhibition or blockade of negative feedback mechanisms. The neurotransmitters affected are predominantly serotonin and noradrenaline, although certain medicines modulate the effects of melatonin and to a lesser extent dopamine. Whilst antidepressants affect neurotransmitters and their receptors at the synaptic level, their therapeutic effects may be mediated through broader changes in the functioning of neuronal pathways and the activity of specific brain regions. The adverse effects of antidepressants result from increased levels of neurotransmitters and through blockade of a variety of neurotransmitter receptors (e.g. muscarinic, serotonergic, alpha-adrenergic).

Rapid Medicines Management for Healthcare Professionals, First Edition. Paul Deslandes, Simon Young and Ben Pitcher.
© 2020 John Wiley & Sons Ltd. Published 2020 by John Wiley & Sons Ltd.

What's the difference between different types?

Antidepressants from different groups exert their effects in different ways. Whilst there is limited evidence to indicate that one medicine or group of medicines is more effective than another, adverse effects vary, reflecting pharmacodynamic differences. The TCAs have greater toxicity (particularly in overdose), whilst MAOIs are associated with potentially dangerous interactions with certain medicines and foods, and for this reason their use has been largely superseded by SSRIs, SNRIs, and mirtazapine.

How are these drugs given?

Regularly (usually daily or twice a day), by mouth, on a long-term basis to treat chronic illness.

Dosing

SSRIs, SNRIs, and mirtazapine can be initiated at treatment doses. This may be an advantage, as it can take one or two weeks for the therapeutic effect of antidepressants to become apparent (longer in the elderly).

TCAs must be initiated at a low dose and gradually titrated upwards to minimise the risk of adverse effects (in particular sedation and postural hypotension).

What are the notable adverse effects to look out for?

Hyponatraemia may occur with all antidepressants and is more common in the elderly.

Serotonin syndrome (characterised by autonomic changes, confusion, and muscular rigidity) has been reported, particularly when medicines that increase levels of serotonin (e.g. SSRIs, MAOIs, tramadol) are given in combination or when taken in overdose. This is a rare condition but may nevertheless be life-threatening and requires emergency treatment.

SSRIs. Nausea, vomiting, agitation, and anxiety can occur early in treatment (this usually wears off after 10–14 days). Sexual dysfunction is an ongoing problem and may affect patient concordance. Also diarrhoea, insomnia, and drowsiness.

SNRIs. As with SSRIs, but also include sweating, tachycardia, palpitations, dry mouth, and constipation.

Mirtazapine. Sedation, increased appetite, and weight gain.

TCAs. Antimuscarinic effects (blurred vision, dry mouth, constipation, urinary retention), sedation, and weight gain are common.

MAOIs. Drowsiness, antimuscarinic effects (blurred vision, dry mouth, constipation, urinary retention) and insomnia are the most common adverse effects. Headache can occur and is also a possible sign of a dangerous interaction with tyramine-containing foods and sympathomimetic agents (see below).

How can the adverse effects be minimised?

SSRIs. Insomnia or drowsiness may be minimised by administering the dose in the morning or evening. Sexual dysfunction may require switching to a different antidepressant (e.g. mirtazapine).

Mirtazapine. Sedation may improve as the dose is increased. Weight gain may respond to dietary advice.

TCAs, A gradual dose titration helps to reduce the side effects on initiation. Lifestyle and dietary advice may help to minimise constipation and weight gain. If this is ineffective, laxatives may be prescribed for constipation.

What drug interactions are important?

Hyponatraemia may lead to increases in lithium levels, leading to lithium toxicity.

Combinations of medicines which increase levels of serotonin (see the section on adverse effects).

SSRIs and SNRIs may increase the risk of bleeding, particularly in combination with non-steroidal anti-inflammatory drugs, antiplatelet drugs, and warfarin.

The SSRIs fluoxetine, fluvoxamine, and paroxetine are inhibitors of cytochrome P450 enzymes and are therefore associated with pharmacokinetic interactions. Caution is required, particularly in combination with drugs with narrow therapeutic ranges (e.g. phenytoin, clozapine, and TCAs).

TCAs. Other antimuscarinic medicines (e.g. procyclidine, diphenhydramine) will increase the risk of urinary retention, constipation etc. Other sedative medicines will increase the risk of drowsiness. Many TCAs are metabolised via CYP2D6 enzymes; any drugs inhibiting the effects of these enzymes (e.g. cimetidine, duloxetine, some SSRIs) may increase the risk of adverse effects of TCAs.

MAOIs. Consumption of foods rich in tyramine (e.g. cheeses, liver pate, and yeast and meat extracts) and sympathomimetic medicines (e.g. ephedrine and pseudoephedrine, which are available over the counter from pharmacies often as ingredients in cough and cold remedies) can result in hypertensive crisis. Patients should carry a treatment card advising that they are taking an MAOI and be advised about the seriousness of this interaction. The use of other antidepressants as well as other medicines which increase neurotransmitter levels should generally be avoided in combination with MAOIs.

Discontinuing treatment

Relapse following antidepressant discontinuation is common and treatment should normally be continued for a minimum of six months after resolution of symptoms (longer after repeated episodes of depression).

When discontinuing, the dose is normally reduced gradually before stopping to minimise the risk of withdrawal effects , although there is limited evidence to support this approach. Withdrawal effects are a significant concern, may be prolonged, and may be particularly problematic with shorter acting medicines such as paroxetine and venlafaxine.

When switching from one antidepressant to another (due to adverse effects or lack of effect), a cross-tapering approach is commonly used whereby the dose of the first medicine is gradually reduced as the dose of the second medicine is gradually increased. This approach is not always appropriate, particularly when switching from fluoxetine (which has a long-acting metabolite) and in switches involving MAOIs (increased risk of serotonin syndrome). Specialist advice should be obtained.

51 Benzodiazepines and Z-Drugs

Benzodiazepines are used to treat a number of conditions and are typically grouped according to their usual indication. However, there may be some overlap across the groups, with individual medicines used for more than one indication.

Commonly used examples

Benzodiazepine anxiolytics. Chlordiazepoxide (Librium®), diazepam (Valium®), lorazepam (Ativan®), oxazepam. Others such as alprazolam and flunitrazepam are not prescribable on the NHS in the UK.

Benzodiazepine hypnotics. Lormetazepam, nitrazepam (Mogadon®), temazepam.

Benzodiazepine other. Clobazam, clonazepam, midazolam.

'Z-drug' hypnotics. Zaleplon, zolpidem, zopiclone.

Are these drugs all the same?

Benzodiazepines and Z-drugs all have similar (but not identical) mechanisms of action, but may be used for different indications, usually depending upon their onset and duration of action.

What are these drugs used to treat?

Benzodiazepines. Short-term treatment of anxiety and insomnia. They are also used as adjunctive therapy in the treatment of epilepsy, as muscle relaxants, for pre-operative sedation, for acute agitation, and in alcohol withdrawal.

Z drugs. Short-term treatment of insomnia.

What do these drugs do?

Benzodiazepines and Z-drugs are agonists at the benzodiazepine receptor binding site of the $GABA_A$ receptor. The $GABA_A$ receptor is a chloride channel that is opened in response to the binding of the neurotransmitter gamma-amino butyric acid (GABA). Opening of the channel results in an influx of chloride ions into the neuron, which results in hyperpolarisation and a reduction in excitability. GABA is therefore termed an inhibitory transmitter as it reduces neuronal firing and the excitability of the central nervous system. Binding of benzodiazepines and Z-drugs to the benzodiazepine receptor potentiates the effects of GABA, enhancing its inhibitory effects. This results in suppression of the central nervous system, leading to sedative, anticonvulsant, and other effects.

Rapid Medicines Management for Healthcare Professionals, First Edition. Paul Deslandes, Simon Young and Ben Pitcher.
© 2020 John Wiley & Sons Ltd. Published 2020 by John Wiley & Sons Ltd.

What's the difference between benzodiazepines and Z-drugs?

The pharmacodynamic properties of the benzodiazepines and Z-drugs are broadly similar, but the different medicines have differing pharmacokinetic properties. Benzodiazepines may have rapid (diazepam) or slower (oxazepam) onset of action due to their lipid solubility. Their durations of action also vary, with longer-acting agents (such as diazepam and chlordiazepoxide) having active metabolites. Z-drugs are typically fast acting with a relatively short duration, reducing the incidence of next-day sedation. Zaleplon achieves peak plasma levels within one to two hours (useful in reducing time to sleep onset), but the short duration of action may not help patients with night-time waking.

How are these drugs given?

Regularly (up to four times a day), by mouth, on a short-term basis to treat anxiety or insomnia.

As required, by mouth or intramuscular injection on a short-term basis to treat acute behavioural disturbance associated with mental illness.

Regularly (up to four times a day), by mouth for epilepsy.

As required by mouth in response to symptoms of alcohol withdrawal.

Acutely buccally, by intravenous injection or rectally to treat prolonged seizures.

Acutely parenterally prior to anaesthesia.

Dosing

As with many medicines, initiate at a low dose and gradually titrate upwards as required. Due to pharmacokinetic changes, the effects of benzodiazepines may be more pronounced in the elderly, and dose adjustment may be necessary to help to minimise the risk of serious adverse effects such as falls.

What are the notable adverse effects to look out for?

Benzodiazepines and Z-drugs are safer than the older barbiturate-type sedatives which they have largely replaced. Nevertheless, tolerance to some of their effects and withdrawal symptoms on discontinuation can develop. These may be signs of developing dependence and specialist advice should be sought. Memory loss, disinhibition, and sedation are possible adverse effects.

How can the adverse effects be minimised?

The use of short-term treatment or as required short courses may help to minimise the risk of dependence compared to continued use on a longer-term basis.

The acute effects of benzodiazepine overdose can be reversed using the $GABA_A$ receptor antagonist flumazenil.

What drug interactions are important?

Combining benzodiazepines with other sedatives (including alcohol) can increase their sedative and other effects.

Discontinuing treatment

When discontinuing treatment, the dose of benzodiazepine should normally be reduced gradually to minimise the risk of withdrawal symptoms. Withdrawal effects are more common with shorter-acting benzodiazepines and some patients may prefer to switch to a longer-acting medicine (e.g. diazepam) when discontinuing, although this is not always the case and patient preference should be considered. Not all patients will experience withdrawal effects, but if they do occur they may continue for several weeks and may resemble and be mistaken for symptoms of the underlying anxiety disorder.

52 Dopamine-enhancing Drugs

A number of physiological processes are controlled by the neurotransmitter dopamine acting via specific dopamine receptors. Dopamine-enhancing drugs are used to treat conditions where increased levels of dopamine or an increased effect of dopamine is required, the most common of which is Parkinson's disease.

Commonly used examples

Dopamine precursors. Levodopa (given as benserazide/levodopa or carbidopa/levodopa combination products).

Dopamine receptor agonists. Apomorphine, bromocriptine, cabergoline, pergolide, pramipexole, ropinirole, rotigotine.

Enzyme inhibitors. Entacapone, tolcapone, rasagiline, selegiline.

Are these drugs all the same?

This group of medicines all increase the effects of dopamine in the brain. However, they do this through different pharmacodynamic mechanisms and some are used to treat a number of different conditions.

What are these drugs used to treat?

Parkinson's disease.
Hyperprolactinaemia.
Restless legs syndrome.
Acromegaly.

What do these drugs do?

Parkinson's disease is characterised by a loss of dopaminergic neurons in brain pathways involved with co-ordinating movement. Medicines used to treat this disorder cannot reverse the underlying neuronal loss but instead attempt to address the resulting reduction in dopaminergic function. They do this through a variety of mechanisms, including increasing the amount of dopamine available by providing the precursor chemical or inhibiting metabolic enzymatic degradation of dopamine. Alternatively, medicines may directly stimulate dopamine receptors.

Prolactin is a hormone best known for its role in enabling mammals, usually females, to produce milk. Release of prolactin from the pituitary gland is inhibited by the action of the neurotransmitter dopamine. By stimulating dopamine receptors (thus mimicking the effect of dopamine), dopamine receptor agonists reduce prolactin release.

Rapid Medicines Management for Healthcare Professionals, First Edition. Paul Deslandes, Simon Young and Ben Pitcher.
© 2020 John Wiley & Sons Ltd. Published 2020 by John Wiley & Sons Ltd.

What's the difference between different types?

Dopamine precursors deliver levodopa to the brain, which is metabolised in neurons to dopamine, therefore increasing the amount of dopamine available to act as a neurotransmitter. Levodopa is formulated as a combination product (typically with carbidopa or benserazide). These additional components are inhibitors of the enzyme dopa-decarboxylase and prevent the conversion of levodopa to dopamine in the body before it enters the brain. This allows a smaller amount of levodopa to be given, reducing the risks of adverse effects.

Dopamine agonists directly stimulate dopamine receptors, mimicking the effect of endogenous dopamine. They can be grouped according to whether or not they are derived from the ergot fungus. Those that are not ergot derived (e.g. ropinirole) are better tolerated and are therefore generally used in preference to ergot-derived drugs (e.g. bromocriptine).

The enzyme inhibitors inhibit the action of one of two enzymes responsible for different aspects of dopamine degradation in the brain. The enzymes are monoamine oxidase B (MAO-B), inhibited by rasagiline and selegilline, and catechol-o-methyl transferase (COMT), inhibited by entacapone and tolcapone. Inhibition of these enzymes increases the amount of dopamine available to act as a neurotransmitter.

How are these drugs given?
Dopamine precursors
Regularly (usually three or four times a day, but may be less frequently as modified-release preparations), by mouth, on a long-term basis for Parkinson's disease.

Levodopa may also be administered in combination with carbidopa as an intra-duodenal gel (Duodopa®).

Dopamine agonists
Regularly (usually daily or twice a day, but may be more frequently depending upon the medicine), by mouth, on a long-term basis for Parkinson's disease.

Regularly, daily, transdermally as an adhesive patch, on a long-term basis for Parkinson's disease.

Apomorphine is given by subcutaneous injection under specialist supervision.

Enzyme inhibitors
MAO-B inhibitors. Regularly, usually daily, by mouth, on a long-term basis for Parkinson's disease.

COMT inhibitors. Regularly, at the same time as levodopa preparations, by mouth, on a long-term basis for Parkinson's disease.

Dosing
As with many medicines, initiate at a low dose and gradually titrate upwards.

Modified-release levodopa preparations (such as Sinemet CR®) or more frequent dosing of immediate-release levodopa preparations may be used as the disease progresses in an attempt to reduce 'off' periods where the patient suffers from rigidity and freezing towards the end of the dosing period. Dosing of these medicines may be individualised and medicines administration may need to occur at precise times.

What are the notable adverse effects to look out for?

Increased dopaminergic activity in the vomiting centre of the brain may lead to nausea and vomiting.

Daytime sleepiness may result from increased dopaminergic activity, but may also be related to symptoms of Parkinson's disease.

Due to the association between increased dopaminergic activity and positive symptoms of psychosis, patients may experience hallucinations and delusions when treated with dopamine-enhancing medicines.

Dopamine agonists may lead to impulsive behaviours, such as gambling and binge eating in some patients.

How can the adverse effects be minimised?

A slow dose titration of the dopamine-enhancing medicine may help to address side effects.

Nausea and vomiting can be managed with peripherally acting dopamine antagonists such as domperidone.

Daytime sleepiness should be assessed to identify and resolve any underlying cause.

Symptoms of psychosis may be managed with small doses of the antipsychotics quetiapine or clozapine.

Patients should be advised of the risk of impulse control disorders associated with dopamine agonists.

What needs to be monitored?

Response to treatment and adverse effects.

What drug interactions are important?

Drugs that inhibit the effects of dopamine (e.g. antipsychotics and metoclopramide) reduce the effectiveness of dopamine-enhancing drugs.

Levodopa and dopamine agonists may be associated with hypotension and other drugs causing hypotension (e.g. beta-blockers and angiotensin converting enzyme inhibitors) will increase this effect.

Administration of monoamine oxidase type A (MAO-A) inhibitor antidepressants (e.g. phenelzine) in combination with levodopa may result in hypertensive crisis and should be avoided. This effect may also be seen when MAO-A inhibitors are used in combination with COMT inhibitors (e.g. entacapone) and MAO-B inhibitors (e.g. selegiline), and these combinations should also be avoided.

Discontinuing treatment

If reducing or discontinuing treatment, the dose of dopamine-enhancing medicines should normally be reduced gradually before stopping to minimise the risk of withdrawal symptoms, including neuroleptic malignant syndrome.

53 Lithium

Brand names include Priadel®, Camcolit®, Liskonum®, Li Liquid®.

What is lithium?

Lithium has been used in the treatment of psychiatric disorders for over 100 years. Chemically, lithium ions are similar to sodium ions and as a result the body treats the two elements in similar ways (particularly with regards to elimination via the kidney).

What is lithium used to treat?

Treatment and prophylaxis of mania, bipolar disorder, and recurrent depression.
Treatment and prophylaxis of aggressive or self-harming behaviour.

What does lithium do?

Symptoms of bipolar disorder and depression are believed to be associated with changes in neuronal activity in certain brain regions. Lithium is effective in reducing the risk of episodes of both manic and depressive relapse in bipolar disorder. It is also known to significantly reduce the risk of suicide in both bipolar disorder and major depression. The actions of lithium at a cellular level are not fully understood. It may affect neurotransmitter function and intracellular signalling

How is lithium given?

Regularly, by mouth, on a long-term basis to treat chronic mental illness.
Tablets are typically formulated as modified-release preparations of lithium carbonate and are usually given once a day. Different tablets have different pharmacokinetic properties, therefore patients should be maintained on the same preparation and caution is required if switching between preparations.
Liquid preparations contain lithium citrate and are usually given twice a day. Lithium carbonate and lithium citrate do not contain the same amounts of elemental lithium, therefore dose adjustment may be required when switching between tablet and liquid formulations.

Dosing

Lithium has a narrow therapeutic range, therefore careful dosing is required. A low starting dose, such as 400 mg daily of Priadel® (lower in the elderly), is typically used with subsequent dose increases according to response. Regular plasma level monitoring is required with samples taken 12 hours post dose. The therapeutic plasma level is typically

Rapid Medicines Management for Healthcare Professionals, First Edition. Paul Deslandes, Simon Young and Ben Pitcher.
© 2020 John Wiley & Sons Ltd. Published 2020 by John Wiley & Sons Ltd.

$0.4–1\,mmol\,l^{-1}$, although the response of individual patients will vary and the level required is also related to the illness being treated.

Continuation of lithium treatment is very important in optimising outcome. Patients should be advised prior to initiation of the need to continue treatment for prolonged periods.

What are the notable adverse effects to look out for?

Lithium may be associated with potentially life-threatening toxicity and requires careful therapeutic drug monitoring. Signs of toxicity include a coarse tremor, gastrointestinal (GI) disturbance, muscle weakness, drowsiness and ataxia, and in severe cases convulsions, coma, and death.

Adverse effects are generally dose related and increase in severity with increasing plasma level. Common adverse effects include a fine tremor, GI disturbance (diarrhoea, metallic taste, nausea), polydipsia, polyuria, hypothyroidism, and weight gain. Lithium can also reduce renal function and may cause hyperparathyroidism.

Lithium has been associated with the foetal cardiac abnormality known as Ebstein's anomaly. As a result, the use of lithium during pregnancy requires careful consideration of the possible risks and benefits.

How can the adverse effects be minimised?

Hypothyroidism is commonly treated with levothyroxine tablets. Tremor may be treated with propranolol.

A healthy diet and lifestyle will help to minimise weight gain.

What needs to be monitored?

Lithium plasma levels should be checked following initiation and after any dose change (usually five to seven days post initiation or dose change). Once stabilised, plasma levels should be checked every three months for the first year of treatment, then every three to six months depending upon the patient.

Lithium therapy can affect the thyroid gland and renal function. Regular thyroid function tests and estimated glomerular filtration rate (eGFR) are required prior to treatment and at six-monthly intervals during treatment (eGFR will be monitored more frequently if renal function is reduced). Weight and serum electrolytes should also be monitored prior to initiation and at six-monthly intervals. Calcium monitoring is important due to the risk of hyperparathyroidism.

The patient will have a 'Purple Book' (Lithium Therapy Pack, including a monitoring record book) that records monitoring, provides information to care providers, etc.

Other recommended monitoring: Electrocardiogram at baseline particularly in patients with risk factors for, or established, cardiovascular disease.

What drug interactions are important?

Because lithium is renally excreted, medicines which affect the functioning of the kidney can increase lithium plasma levels with the potential to cause toxicity. Examples include non-steroidal anti-inflammatory drugs, diuretics (especially thiazide type), and angiotensin converting enzyme inhibitors.

Lithium plasma concentration is influenced by sodium concentration. Any conditions (e.g. dehydration, vomiting, diarrhoea, change to a low salt diet) or medications (e.g. antidepressants, carbamazepine) causing hyponatraemia may lead to increased lithium plasma levels.

There are a number of isolated reports of neurotoxicity when lithium has been given in combination with other central nervous system active medicines. Due to the narrow therapeutic range of lithium, patients should be aware of the signs of toxicity and told to report any adverse effects.

Discontinuing treatment

Discontinuation of lithium therapy is associated with a high risk of relapse. If withdrawal is necessary, a gradual dose reduction over at least four weeks (and preferably longer) is advised. However, relapse may still occur despite a gradual dose reduction, and this should be a consideration when making any prescribing decisions.

54 Drugs for Dementia

Commonly used examples
Cholinesterase inhibitors. Donepezil (Aricept®), galantamine, rivastigmine.
Other. Memantine.

Are these drugs all the same?
Antidementia medicines can be grouped according to their mechanisms of action and the severity of disease for which they are used to treat.

What are these drugs used to treat?
Cholinesterase inhibitors. Mild to moderate Alzheimer's disease.
Memantine. Moderate to severe Alzheimer's disease.

What do these drugs do?
Symptoms of dementia result from neurodegenerative processes occurring in the brain. Neuronal cell death results in symptoms of cognitive impairment and memory loss. Different pathophysiological processes underlie different types of dementia. The most common type is Alzheimer's disease and the antidementia drugs are licensed in this disorder (although they are sometimes used in other types of dementia). However, none of the medicines that are currently available to treat dementia reverse the disease process; instead they attempt to improve signs and symptoms, and reduce neurotoxicity. Disease-modifying and preventative medicines may become available in the future. Current therapy aims to improve cognition and memory through enhancement of cholinergic neurotransmitter systems in the brain or to limit the neurotoxicity associated with the activity of the excitatory neurotransmitter glutamate. Antidementia drugs may help to reduce behavioural and psychological symptoms of certain types of dementia, although the evidence base for this is somewhat limited.

What's the difference between different types?
The function of the neurotransmitter acetylcholine in certain brain pathways is important in the development of memory. The action of acetylcholine is rapidly terminated by the enzyme acetylcholinesterase, which metabolises and inactivates it. The cholinesterase inhibitor group of medicines inhibits the enzyme responsible for the metabolism of acetylcholine, prolonging the effect of the neurotransmitter and improving memory. Each of the cholinesterase inhibitor medicines (donepezil, galantamine, and rivastigmine) has slightly different pharmacodynamic properties, but there appears to be little evidence of a difference in therapeutic effectiveness between them.

Rapid Medicines Management for Healthcare Professionals, First Edition. Paul Deslandes, Simon Young and Ben Pitcher.
© 2020 John Wiley & Sons Ltd. Published 2020 by John Wiley & Sons Ltd.

The *N*-methyl D-aspartate (NMDA) receptor mediates some of the effects of the excitatory amino acid neurotransmitter glutamate. Stimulation of NMDA receptors by glutamate mediates calcium influx into neurons, resulting in neuronal excitation. However, prolonged stimulation can result in neuronal death. Memantine is an NMDA receptor antagonist and inhibits some of the neurotoxic effects of glutamate, resulting in reduced neuronal loss with some evidence of enhanced cognitive functioning.

How are these drugs given?

Regularly (once or twice a day), by mouth, on a long-term basis for symptoms of dementia.

Regularly, transdermally (via adhesive patches), on a long-term basis for symptoms of dementia.

Dosing

Initiate at a low dose and gradually titrate upwards. The full therapeutic effect may take some weeks to develop.

Dosing may need to be adjusted or the medicine may be contraindicated depending on renal or hepatic function. This will depend on the medicine prescribed. For example, galantamine requires dosage adjustment in certain severities of hepatic and renal impairment, and memantine requires dosage adjustment in certain severities of renal impairment. Further information for all of these medicines in relation to patients with renal or hepatic impairment should be obtained from the relevant summary of product characteristics.

What are the notable adverse effects to look out for?

Acetylcholine is the neurotransmitter responsible for mediating the physiological effects of the parasympathetic nervous system. Some of these effects include increased gastrointestinal motility and reduced cardiac output. The cholinesterase inhibitors enhance the effects of acetylcholine and may therefore cause adverse effects such as diarrhoea, urinary incontinence, and bradycardia related to increased parasympathetic activity.

Memantine may cause dyspnoea (shortness of breath), which may require medical treatment.

How can the adverse effects be minimised?

A gradual dose titration with regular assessment of adverse effects may help to improve tolerability.

What needs to be monitored?

Cognitive function is typically checked at regular intervals to assess response to treatment. The patient's tolerance of the treatment will also guide dosing.

What drug interactions are important?

Medicines affecting the action of the neurotransmitter acetylcholine may enhance or inhibit the effects of cholinesterase inhibitors. In particular, medicines that antagonise the effects of acetylcholine at its muscarinic receptors have been associated with confusion and cognitive impairment in the elderly. Drugs used for their antimuscarinic effects include atropine, hyoscine, orphenadrine, procyclidine, trihexyphenidyl, and certain drugs used for urinary incontinence (e.g. oxybutynin), and all of these may be associated with worsening cognitive impairment. In addition to the above, many medicines are associated with antimuscarinic properties as a side effect. These include tricyclic antidepressants (e.g. amitriptyline, clomipramine), certain antipsychotics (e.g. chlorpromazine, clozapine, promethazine), and certain antihistamines (e.g. alimemazine, clemastine) (note that these lists are not exhaustive).

The neurotransmitter acetylcholine has effects on the heart (causing bradycardia). Cholinesterase inhibitors increase the effect of acetylcholine and may therefore enhance the bradycardia caused by certain calcium channel blockers (e.g. verapamil), beta-blockers (e.g. propranolol), and digoxin.

Galantamine is metabolised through the cytochrome P450 enzyme system. Medicines inhibiting these enzymes (e.g. paroxetine, ketoconazole) may increase plasma levels, which may lead to an increased risk of adverse effects.

Memantine may enhance the effects of medicines such as amantadine and ketamine due to their similar effects on NMDA receptors. Memantine may also increase the effects of dopaminergic (e.g. levodopa) and anticholinergic (e.g. procyclidine) medicines.

Discontinuing treatment

Treatment with antidementia drugs is typically ongoing, on a long–term basis, and should not necessarily be stopped due to increasing symptom severity. Treatment may be discontinued due to poor tolerability (adverse effects) or if the patient is no longer deemed to be deriving any benefit from the medicine. Switching from one cholinesterase inhibitor to another may be of benefit where there is poor tolerability or poor response.

55 Anticonvulsants

A significant number of medicines are available to prevent and treat epileptic seizures, many of which are also used for a number of other indications. Some of those that are prescribed more commonly are discussed below. For further information relating to benzodiazepines, please refer to Chapter 51, which describes these medicines.

Commonly used examples

Benzodiazepines (e.g. midazolam), carbamazepine, oxcarbazepine, gabapentin, pregabalin, lamotrigine, levetiracetam, phenytoin, topiramate, and valproate (sodium valproate, valproic acid).

Are these drugs all the same?

Antiepileptics are a diverse group of medicines with a broad range of pharmacodynamic and pharmacokinetic properties. Different medicines may be associated with a number of potentially serious adverse effects and drug interactions, making their management complex.

What are these drugs used to treat?

Epilepsy. The choice of medicine will vary with the type of epilepsy as well as individual patient factors. In focal epilepsy, lamotrigine, carbamazepine, topiramate, or oxcarbazepine are commonly used; in generalised epilepsy valproate, topiramate, or lamotrigine are commonly used.

Mood disorders. Valproate is commonly used as a mood stabiliser in the treatment of bipolar affective disorder. Other antiepileptic medicines, including carbamazepine, lamotrigine, and topiramate, may also be used as mood stabilisers.

Neuropathic pain. Carbamazepine, gabapentin and pregabalin.

As an adjunct in alcohol withdrawal. Carbamazepine and oxcarbazepine.

What do these drugs do?

Epileptic seizures result from abnormal, spontaneous, excitatory neuronal activity (increased neuronal activation and firing). Antiepileptic medicines reduce the level of excitation in the brain through different mechanisms, which include interactions with ion channels (sodium or calcium) located in neuronal membranes, by potentiating the effects of inhibitory neurotransmitters (e.g. gamma-aminobutyric acid, GABA) or reducing the effects of excitatory neurotransmitters (e.g. glutamate) or a combination of one or more mechanisms.

Rapid Medicines Management for Healthcare Professionals, First Edition. Paul Deslandes, Simon Young and Ben Pitcher.
© 2020 John Wiley & Sons Ltd. Published 2020 by John Wiley & Sons Ltd.

What's the difference between different types?

Antiepileptic medicines vary in their mechanisms of action and the precise pharmacodynamic properties of several of these drugs remain unclear.

Carbamazepine and oxcarbazepine. These drugs are structurally related and appear to act by stabilising sodium channels and in the case of carbamazepine by reducing glutamate release. Carbamazepine is an inducer of CYP450 enzymes, resulting in many drug interactions. Oxcarbazepine is a weak CYP450 enzyme inducer and also inhibits CYP2C19.

Gabapentin and pregabalin. Both of these drugs bind to neuronal calcium channels, reducing excitatory neurotransmitter release.

Lamotrigine. Reduces the release of the excitatory neurotransmitter glutamate and inhibits sodium channels.

Levetiracetam. Has an effect on neuronal calcium levels and may alter neurotransmitter release.

Phenytoin. Has multiple pharmacodynamic effects, including reduction of sodium conductance and neurotransmitter release, and increased post-synaptic GABAergic neurotransmission. Phenytoin is both an inducer of, and is metabolised by, CYP450 enzymes, resulting in a number of drug interactions.

Valproate. Enhances the effects of the inhibitory neurotransmitter GABA.

How are these drugs given?

Regularly (usually daily or twice a day, but may be more frequently depending upon the medicine and formulation), by mouth, on a long-term basis as maintenance therapy.

Regularly, by mouth, on a short-term basis as adjunctive treatment to prevent a seizure.

As required, sublingually, rectally or by injection on a short-term basis to treat acute seizures.

Regularly, by mouth, on a long-term basis to treat mood disorders or neuropathic pain.

Note: Due to pharmacokinetic variation between different manufacturers' brands of the same medicine and the risk of seizures due to fluctuating plasma levels, patients should not be switched between brands of carbamazepine, phenytoin, phenobarbital, and primidone. For other antiepileptics, including valproate, lamotrigine, perampanel, retigabine, rufinamide, clobazam, clonazepam, oxcarbazepine, eslicarbazepine, zonisamide, and topiramate, caution is required if patients are switched between different brands of the same medicine.

Dosing

As with many medicines, initiate at a low dose and gradually titrate upwards to minimise the risk of adverse effects. Some antiepileptic medicines may themselves worsen seizure control initially.

Carbamazepine and phenytoin have complex pharmacokinetics and narrow therapeutic ranges, necessitating caution in dosing and careful monitoring for signs of adverse effects. Carbamazepine is an inducer of the hepatic cytochrome P450 enzyme system and induces its own metabolism, resulting in a prolonged period to reach steady-state levels. Dosage adjustment should not be considered until steady state is reached, normally after approximately two weeks of treatment. Phenytoin is also a CYP450 inducer and has non-linear pharmacokinetics whereby a small increase in dose may be associated with a significant increase in plasma levels that may result in toxicity – careful dosing is required.

What are the notable adverse effects to look out for?

Foetal abnormalities. Valproate use during pregnancy is associated with a high risk of congenital abnormalities and neurodevelopmental disorders in childhood. As a result, its use should usually be avoided in female children and adolescents, and women of childbearing potential. Carbamazepine, phenytoin, and phenobarbital are hepatic enzyme inducers and increase folate metabolism, thereby increasing the risk of congenital abnormalities when these medicines are used in pregnancy. Lamotrigine and topiramate have also been associated with foetal abnormalities.

Rash. A number of antiepileptic medicines (most notably lamotrigine and carbamazepine) have been associated with an increased risk of serious rash (Stevens–Johnson syndrome and toxic epidermal necrolysis), which may be fatal.

Blood and hepatic disorders. Several antiepileptic medicines are associated with blood or liver disorders, including valproate, carbamazepine, phenytoin, and lamotrigine.

Vitamin D deficiency. Hepatic enzyme inducers (e.g. carbamazepine).

Misuse potential. Gabapentin and particularly pregabalin are recognised as having abuse potential and are associated with euphoria, relaxation, and other psychotropic effects.

Carbamazepine and phenytoin toxicity. Signs include diplopia, dizziness, and gastrointestinal disturbance (carbamazepine), dysarthria and nystagmus (phenytoin), and ataxia (both).

How can the adverse effects be minimised?

Modified-release preparations can be used to improve tolerability and allow once-daily dosing of many antiepileptic medicines.

Foetal abnormalities. Women should be advised of the risks and benefits of taking antiepileptic medication during pregnancy prior to treatment. Specialist advice should be obtained for women wishing to become or who have become pregnant whilst taking antiepileptic medication.

Rash. Slow dose titration is important to reduce the risk of lamotrigine-induced rash. Stevens–Johnson syndrome associated with carbamazepine and phenytoin is more common in people of Han Chinese and Thai origin. A genetic test is available to identify those most at risk prior to treatment initiation. If rash occurs, treatment should be discontinued immediately.

Blood disorders. Patients should be advised to observe for bruising, sore throat, fever, and other signs of bone marrow suppression.

What needs to be monitored?

The nature and frequency of monitoring will depend upon the specific medicine, but may include liver function tests, full blood count, and urea and electrolytes.

Medicine plasma levels – therapeutic drug monitoring may be useful in certain circumstances (e.g. to give an indication of medication adherence or to investigate possible toxicity), but typically is not routinely recommended.

What drug interactions are important?

Carbamazepine, phenytoin, and the barbiturate phenobarbital are all potent hepatic cytochrome P450 enzyme inducers. This may result in a reduction in the plasma levels of a number of other medicines with the potential to result in treatment failure.

Concomitant use of drugs increasing the levels of carbamazepine and phenytoin (e.g. the hepatic enzyme inhibitor erythromycin) may result in potential toxicity.

Drugs reducing the levels of antiepileptics (e.g. hepatic enzyme inducers such as rifampicin) may increase the risk of seizures.

Medicines reducing the seizure threshold (e.g. bupropion, clozapine) may increase the risk of seizures.

Carbamazepine may cause hyponatraemia, which may lead to increased lithium levels (and may result in lithium toxicity). It may also cause bone marrow suppression and increase the risk of agranulocytosis with medicines such as clozapine.

Discontinuing treatment

The usual aim of treatment for epilepsy is to reduce seizure frequency, preferably with monotherapy, in order to reduce the risk of adverse effects. If an initial treatment titrated to the maximum tolerated dose is ineffective, and it is necessary to switch between medicines, the new treatment is typically titrated to an effective dose before the dose of the original medicine is gradually reduced and then stopped.

When discontinuing treatment, the dose of antiepileptic should normally be reduced gradually (over at least four weeks) before stopping to reduce the risk of withdrawal related seizures. Withdrawal of treatment requires specialist management with the full engagement of the patient.

56 Drugs for Alcohol Withdrawal

Sometimes called 'detox' or Clinical Institute Withdrawal Assessment for Alcohol (CIWA, pronounced 'see-wah').

Alcohol dependence is characterised by 'craving, tolerance, a preoccupation with alcohol, and continued drinking despite harmful consequences'. Alcohol dependence describes a strong and frequently uncontrollable desire to drink. Many factors are considered in diagnosing alcohol dependence. However, a score of 20 or greater in the Alcohol Use Disorders Identification Test (AUDIT) indicates alcohol dependence, whilst the Severity of Alcohol Dependence Questionnaire (SADQ) indicates the severity of dependence.

An alcohol-dependent patient who suddenly stops drinking (or reduces their drinking significantly) can develop alcohol withdrawal syndrome. Alcohol withdrawal is associated with significant morbidity and mortality if it is not properly managed.

Commonly used examples

Pabrinex® [intravenous (i/v) and intramuscular (i/m)].
Diazepam (and benzodiazepines generally, including chlordiazepoxide and lorazepam).
Oral thiamine.
Oxcarbazepine (or carbamazepine).

What are these drugs used to treat?

All of these drugs are used to manage aspects of alcohol withdrawal. Many have additional uses as follows.

Pabrinex is used to replenish water-soluble vitamins, especially in malabsorption syndromes (i/m and i/v) and in chronic, intermittent dialysis (i/v).

Diazepam is indicated for treating anxiety, muscle spasm, spasticity in cerebral palsy, and as a pre-medication for dental and surgical procedures (see Chapter 51).

Oral thiamine is used for treatment of thiamine deficiency.

Oxcarbazepine and carbamazepine are primarily used for the treatment of epilepsy but may also be used to treat neuropathic pain or mood disorders (see Chapter 55).

What do these drugs do?
Pabrinex® (i/v and i/m)

Pabrinex is an injectable product given via the intramuscular (i/m) or intravenous (i/v) route. The complete formulation contains a mixture of vitamins: thiamine (vitamin B1), riboflavin (vitamin B2), pyridoxine (vitamin B6), nicotinamide (a vitamin B3 family member), ascorbic

Rapid Medicines Management for Healthcare Professionals, First Edition. Paul Deslandes, Simon Young and Ben Pitcher.
© 2020 John Wiley & Sons Ltd. Published 2020 by John Wiley & Sons Ltd.

acid (vitamin C), and glucose (only in the i/v preparation). The purpose of using Pabrinex in alcohol withdrawal is to replenish the body's water-soluble vitamins. A combination of factors associated with alcohol dependency means that these vitamins are not sustained at the correct levels in the body in these patients. The aim of the therapy is to raise the vitamin levels and prevent or treat longer-term issues associated with sustained low vitamin level, such as Wernicke–Korsakoff syndrome.

Diazepam

Diazepam is a member of the benzodiazepine family. The drug is used in alcohol withdrawal to suppress the symptoms of the withdrawal process. The main function of using diazepam is to reduce the risk of seizures that can develop during alcohol withdrawal and to act as a short-term substitute for the alcohol as it slowly leaves the body when drinking discontinues. Diazepam enhances the action of the inhibitory neurotransmitter gamma-aminobutyric acid in the central nervous system.

Oral thiamine

Much like Pabrinex, oral thiamine is used to build up deficient levels of vitamin B1 in the alcohol-dependent patient. Like Pabrinex, oral thiamine is essentially a replacement therapy.

Oxcarbazepine/carbamazepine

One or other of these two anticonvulsants may accompany diazepam to prevent the development of seizures during alcohol withdrawal. They are often used if the patient has a history of misusing other drugs that may increase the likelihood of seizures during the alcohol withdrawal process. They are believed to block voltage-sensitive sodium channels and inhibit neuronal firing.

How are these drugs given?

Pabrinex is given either i/m or i/v. The choice of route is usually dependent on the staff skill mix in the clinical area where the detoxification takes place.

Diazepam, thiamine, oxcarbazepine, and carbamazepine are administered by mouth in tablet or liquid form depending upon the drug.

Dosing

Pabrinex is usually given as a fixed regime at the commencement of alcohol detoxification. The dose administered is a combination of a pair of ampoules (I and II). A dose of one pair of ampoules is administered as soon as consent is given and then one pair is administered twice daily for three days. This regime is often repeated if the patient shows signs and symptoms associated with thiamine deficiency.

Diazepam is often given according to the CIWA-Ar detoxification protocol. This method of detoxification is an alternative to a fixed-dose treatment strategy and should be used only when training has been completed by nursing and medical staff. With this method, patients with overt or suspected alcohol withdrawal are objectively assessed for the presence of significant withdrawal at regular intervals. Severity of withdrawal is assessed using a standardised scale, the CIWA-Ar. If found to have significant alcohol withdrawal, the patient is given a dose of diazepam 20 mg. This procedure of standardised assessment and treatment is repeated every 90 minutes until the patient is no longer in withdrawal and detoxification is complete.

Thiamine is usually dosed at 100 mg two to three times daily. This will continue after detoxification.

Oxcarbazepine is typically dosed at 300 mg twice daily for a duration of 7–14 days. The drug is commenced at the start of detoxification.

What are the notable adverse effects to look out for?

Pabrinex and thiamine have few side effects, but hypersensitivity reactions (especially with Pabrinex) are important to consider.

Diazepam causes drowsiness and patients can become dependent on diazepam.

Oxcarbazepine is commonly reported to cause somnolence, headache, dizziness, diplopia, nausea, vomiting, and fatigue.

How can the adverse effects be minimised?

Appropriate dosing and monitoring can help to minimise the risk of adverse effects.

What needs to be monitored?

Pabrinex. Signs/symptoms of hypersensitivity reactions.

Diazepam. Drowsiness, liver function tests: poor liver function may result in impaired diazepam metabolism.

Oxcarbazepine and carbamazepine may cause hyponatraemia and this should be monitored if the drug is used.

What drug interactions are important?

Diazepam interacts with a range of medication. Many of its interactions relate to drowsiness and the potentiation of drowsiness caused by other medications.

Oxcarbazepine interacts in a potentially hazardous fashion with oestrogens, clopidogrel, perampanel progestogens, antidepressants, antipsychotics, mefloquine, and orlistat.

Carbamazepine is a hepatic cytochrome P450 enzyme inducer that can reduce the levels of many other drugs.

Other considerations

Pabrinex i/m is a large volume (7 ml) – good injection technique is required.

Pabrinex i/m is stored in the refrigerator.

Rectal diazepam and postictal diazepam doses are often written into detoxification medication administration charts.

57 Nicotine Replacement Therapy

Commonly used examples

Nicotine gum
Nicotine lozenges
Nicotine sublingual tablets
Nicotine patches
Nicotine inhalators
E-cigarettes

Are these drugs all the same?

All nicotine replacement therapies (NRTs) are a means of delivering nicotine. The main differences seen are the routes by which the nicotine is delivered. This is typically by transdermal patch, inhalation or orally in the form of sublingual tablets, lozenges, or chewing gum.

What are these drugs used to treat?

NRT is used to satiate cravings of nicotine addiction associated with the addictive nature of smoking. Replacing nicotine and eliminating the inhalation of the more harmful chemicals of smoking is a significant health benefit. This is intended to reduce harm, facilitate quitting or relieve nicotine cravings when in environments where it is not possible to smoke (such as in hospital).

What do these drugs do?

The smoking of tobacco products (or consumption by other means) provides the body with a dose of a variety of chemicals, many of them toxic. One of the more notable chemicals is nicotine, a stimulant that acts on nicotinic cholinergic receptors. These are receptors which normally respond to acetylcholine and are involved in numerous processes in the brain and throughout the body. Nicotine has a higher affinity for the receptors found in the brain than in the peripheral nervous system, which is why at doses seen in smoking (or in NRT) the effects are generally limited to the central nervous system. As the dose is increased, more peripheral receptors are activated, leading to side effects.

What's the difference between different types?

The major difference between types of NRTs is the route of delivery as the differences in pharmacokinetic profile of these routes can provide support for patients in different ways.

Rapid Medicines Management for Healthcare Professionals, First Edition. Paul Deslandes, Simon Young and Ben Pitcher.
© 2020 John Wiley & Sons Ltd. Published 2020 by John Wiley & Sons Ltd.

How are these drugs given?

Nicotine patches provide a consistent and continuous supply of nicotine, but they are unable to provide the delivery of sudden bursts of nicotine (in a way similar to smoking a cigarette). Other routes, such nicotine gum and inhalators, can provide that sudden burst of nicotine to help quell the more acute cravings. The inhalator also helps address some of the habitual aspects of smoking, physically emulating the act of holding a cigarette and putting it the mouth.

Dosing

NRTs are available in variety of dosages to allow the dose of nicotine to be tailored to the normal level of nicotine consumed by the patient. This also allows for the dose of nicotine to be reduced as part of a smoking cessation plan. Delivery options which allow a fast delivery of nicotine and therefore a quick relief from cravings are typically administered on an 'as required' basis, whilst patches are typically applied once a day. Topical patches are available that deliver the dose of nicotine over 16 hours or over 24 hours. These are not necessarily interchangeable.

What are the notable adverse effects to look out for?

Whilst NRT is significantly less harmful than smoking, nicotine is still a stimulant and can have a negative impact on the patient. NRT is capable of producing the same nicotine-related side effects as smoking. As those using NRT are smokers, they have usually developed a tolerance to nicotine. However, if the dose of NRT is too high or if the patient swallows the nicotine they may experience side effects, most notably gastrointestinal disturbances. If the dosage of NRT is too low the patient may experience symptoms of nicotine withdrawal, including anxiety, insomnia, and malaise.

How can the adverse effects be minimised?

Tailoring the delivery method to the needs of the patient may improve treatment effectiveness. Use of patches delivering the dose over 16 hours allows a period with reduced nicotine plasma levels, which may help to minimise sleep disturbance.

What drug interactions are important?

Whilst nicotine itself has few significant interactions, it is still important to consider what drugs the patient may be taking. Tobacco smoke contains chemicals which are enzyme inducers and this means that the effects of cytochrome P450 enzymes responsible for metabolising some drugs can be enhanced. Regular smokers may have had the doses of affected drugs increased to account for this. If a patient switches from smoking tobacco products to NRT then the enzyme effects will no longer be enhanced and the higher dose will no longer be necessary. If the dose is not reduced, then the drug concentration could rise to toxic levels. This is especially important in instances where the drug has a narrow therapeutic range (such as theophylline or clozapine) and the harm resulting from toxicity is great.

Discontinuing treatment

Treatment should obviously be discontinued if the patient returns to smoking. Otherwise the NRT will typically be titrated down as a means of weaning the patient off the nicotine and helping to facilitate smoking cessation. If this is the aim, the patient should continue on the starting dose for two to three months before reducing (this may vary according to the product literature).

Other considerations

In recent years electronic cigarettes have dramatically increased in popularity and can now be seen being used as an alternative method of nicotine delivery. E-cigarettes use a battery-powered heater to vaporise a solution (referred to as a 'juice') of nicotine dissolved in vegetable glycerine or propylene glycol with a flavouring added to make it more palatable. This is then inhaled, delivering the nicotine to the lungs in a similar way to smoking, but without all of the other damaging components of tobacco smoke. Currently, E-cigarettes do not form part of the recommended strategies for smoking cessation, but many smokers have used them reduce the harm caused by smoking and by using progressively lower concentrations of nicotine solution wean themselves off nicotine. Reticence to embrace E-cigarettes as a means of smoking cessation stems from concerns about safety. Current research has indicated that the inhalation of vegetable glycerine or propylene glycol vapour is probably safe (or at least significantly safer than smoking). However, due to their relatively recent widespread use the effects of E-cigarette use on the lungs over a lifetime have not been studied. Furthermore, as the 'juices' are not regulated there are concerns about the purity of the ingredients and the potential toxicity of additives and flavouring. The use of E-cigarettes is typically prohibited where smoking is prohibited, e.g. they cannot be used in a hospital setting.

58 Paracetamol

Commonly used examples
- Paracetamol tablets and suspension
- Co-codamol (paracetamol and codeine) and co-dydramol (paracetamol and dihydrocodeine)
- Paracetamol and caffeine
- Paracetamol and decongestants (e.g. Lemsip®)

Are these drugs all the same?
Paracetamol can be used alone or combined with a range of different drugs, most commonly opioid analgesics, but also ibuprofen, or decongestants. The properties of these products will vary slightly depending on the specific ingredients included in the individual preparation.

How do these drugs work?
The exact mechanism of action of paracetamol is not fully understood. Some theories suggest that it has a similar mechanism of action to non-steroidal anti-inflammatory drugs, inhibiting cyclooxygenase (COX) enzymes. However, paracetamol does not have either the gastric irritation or cardiovascular risks associated with COX-1 or COX-2 inhibitors. Other theories suggest its effect may be mediated by the endocannabinoid pathways, but this has not been clearly proven.

The other ingredients found in combination products work through mechanisms including the opioid system and inhibition of COX enzymes. For further details, see Chapters 59 and 71.

What are these drugs used for?
Paracetamol is effective as a first-line analgesic for the treatment of mild to moderate pain and as an antipyretic to help reduce fever and other flu-like symptoms. The addition of other drugs in combination products may provide additional benefit (such as an anti-inflammatory effect with ibuprofen). However, combination products containing low doses of opioids (e.g. codeine 8 mg) may have little benefit over paracetamol alone, but be associated with additional adverse effects.

How are these drugs given?
Paracetamol is most commonly given orally as tablets, capsules or suspension, and occasionally as a suppository. Paracetamol is also available as an intravenous preparation. By administering paracetamol intravenously it is able to enter the blood supply without passing through the liver (see Chapter 13). As such, more of the drug is available to exert an

Rapid Medicines Management for Healthcare Professionals, First Edition. Paul Deslandes, Simon Young and Ben Pitcher.

effect. Whilst oral paracetamol is generally only indicated in mild to moderate pain, i/v paracetamol can be effective in managing post-operative pain.

Combination products are typically given orally as tablets or capsules. Combination products, including codeine, may include small or larger amounts of this opioid (typically 8 or 30 mg). The lower strength products are available over the counter from pharmacies, whereas the higher strength products are available only on prescription.

Dosing

Typically for an adult, the dose of paracetamol is 1 g (two 500 mg tablets) given every 4–6 hours with a maximum dose of 4 g (four 1 g doses) in 24 hours. It is very important that this maximum dose is not exceeded as paracetamol can become very toxic. It is important to note that whilst you can give doses 4 hours apart, if you did this continuously throughout the day, you could end up giving 6 g (six 1 g doses) in a 24-hour period (an overdose).

Children and patients with low body weight or other co-morbidities will have different dosages and lower daily maximums. The *British National Formulary* or local guidance should always be consulted to check the exact dose for your patient.

What are the notable adverse effects to look out for?

Oral paracetamol is generally well tolerated, although intravenous paracetamol can cause cardiovascular side effects such as flushing and hypotension.

Products that combine paracetamol with other drugs will be associated with the adverse effects of the additional ingredients. This may include constipation with opioids and gastric irritation with ibuprofen.

Paracetamol overdose

Whilst paracetamol is a very safe drug when used correctly it has the potential to be lethal if too much is given. Some paracetamol overdoses are accidental, occurring when a patient takes doses that are too large or too frequent in an attempt to manage pain. Others may be deliberate. Whatever the cause, an overdose of paracetamol may not lead to any observable adverse effects but requires urgent medical attention. The metabolism of paracetamol produces a toxic metabolite that damages the liver and kidneys. Patients who have overdosed on paracetamol may require an infusion of *N*-acetyl cysteine (Parvolex®) to help metabolise the toxic by-product and reduce the risk of organ damage.

How can the adverse effects be minimised?

The risk of overdose can be managed by careful dosing. It is important that the patient is aware that they should not only keep within the recommended dose for the paracetamol product they are taking, but also that they should not combine it with other paracetamol-containing products.

Always check with the patient if they have been taking any over-the-counter medication that contains paracetamol (it is important to remember that cold and flu remedies like *Lemsip*® may contain paracetamol). You should also check that paracetamol containing medications have not been written up on more than one part of a patient's drug chart (e.g. in the regular medication section and in the 'as required' section).

What needs to be monitored?

Doses for children are different and typically calculated by age range. Similarly, adults with very low body mass or with pre-existing hepatic dysfunction must receive lower doses to prevent toxicity.

It is important to be aware of the patient's liver function as pre-existing hepatic dysfunction will reduce the patient's ability to metabolise paracetamol and therefore they should be given less in a 24-hour period.

What drug interactions are important?

Paracetamol itself has very few interactions with other drugs and none which are considered potentially serious. However, due to the wide variety of products that contain paracetamol, its status as a General Sales List medicine (available for purchase from shops), and its diversity of use, there is significant risk of more than one paracetamol-containing product being taken at the same time, risking overdose.

59 Opioids

Opioid analgesics (opioid receptor agonists) are widely used for the treatment of pain and may also be prescribed in the management of addiction. Opioid antagonists are available to reverse the effects of opioid analgesics and are used for the treatment of overdose, to reduce adverse effects, and to reduce injecting behaviour in addiction.

Commonly used examples

Weak agonists. Codeine, dihydrocodeine, tramadol.
Strong agonists. Diamorphine, fentanyl, morphine, methadone, oxycodone, pethidine, tapentadol.
Partial agonist. Buprenorphine.
Antagonists. Naloxone, naltrexone, methylnaltrexone.

Are these drugs all the same?

Opioid analgesics are typically classified according to their effects at opioid receptors and the severity of pain that they are used to treat. The available medicines can be grouped as strong, weak or partial agonists. The strong opioids (e.g. morphine) are schedule 2 controlled drugs, and buprenorphine and tramadol are schedule 3 controlled drugs, each with specific record keeping and prescription writing requirements (see Chapter 77 for further details). Loperamide is an opioid agonist that acts peripherally on the gastrointestinal (GI) tract and therefore does not have analgesic properties.

What are these drugs used to treat?

Opioid analgesics are most commonly used in the treatment of pain. Strong agonists are used to treat moderate to severe pain, weak agonists mild to moderate pain.

Opioids may also be used as maintenance strategies in the treatment of addiction, and for dyspnoea in cardiac and pulmonary conditions.

Loperamide is used to treat diarrhoea.

What do these drugs do?

Painful stimuli are detected by peripheral nociceptive receptors, resulting in the activation of primary afferent neurons, which have their terminals in the dorsal horn of the spinal cord. Stimuli of sufficient intensity activate ascending neuronal pathways, which innervate the brainstem and thalamus area of the brain. Processing of these signals results in the stimulus being perceived as painful. Opioid receptors are found in both the dorsal horn of the spinal cord and in the brain, and stimulation of these receptors (either by endogenous opioid peptides or opioid agonist medicines) attenuates the transmission of painful stimuli

Rapid Medicines Management for Healthcare Professionals, First Edition. Paul Deslandes, Simon Young and Ben Pitcher.
© 2020 John Wiley & Sons Ltd. Published 2020 by John Wiley & Sons Ltd.

and perception of pain, resulting in an analgesic effect. The principal receptor involved in mediating these effects is the mu opioid receptor, and the available medicines act via this receptor.

What's the difference between different types?

Opioid analgesics are differentiated by their ability to stimulate the mu opioid receptor and also by their pharmacokinetic properties. Some of these medicines have additional pharmacodynamic targets.

Codeine and dihydrocodeine. These are weak mu receptor agonists that are used to treat mild to moderate pain. Codeine is metabolised to morphine via CYP450 enzymes in the liver. Genetic variation in these enzymes can lead to some people being ultra-rapid metabolisers. This group will experience increased levels of morphine with the potential for toxicity to occur. Codeine should therefore be avoided in known rapid CYP2D6 metabolisers. Conversely, poor metabolisers may not experience an effective analgesic effect from codeine, as they do not readily convert it to morphine.

Morphine, oxycodone, pethidine, and other strong agonists are used to treat moderate to severe pain.

Tramadol and tapentadol. In addition to their effects at the mu opioid receptor, these medicines inhibit the reuptake of noradrenaline and serotonin from the synaptic cleft. This may contribute to their therapeutic and adverse effects. Like codeine, tramadol is metabolised to a more active metabolite in the liver and should be avoided in known ultra-rapid metabolisers.

Methadone is a strong agonist with complex pharmacokinetic properties and a typically longer half-life than other opioids, allowing once daily dosing. This makes it useful as a maintenance treatment in opioid addiction.

Loperamide does not achieve significant concentrations in the brain, but stimulates opioid receptors in the GI tract, resulting in reduced motility and constipation. It is therefore used as a treatment for diarrhoea.

How are these drugs given?

Orally, on a short-term basis for acute pain. Usually once or twice a day as modified-release preparations, but may be more frequently depending upon the medicine.

Transdermal patch on a short-term basis for acute pain. Every three days (fentanyl) or every seven days (buprenorphine).

Short-acting injection. Up to six times a day for acute pain.

Syringe driver subcutaneously for the management of pain in palliative care.

The use of opioid analgesics to treat chronic non-cancer pain is an area of concern due to the safety risks and limited evidence of efficacy.

Dosing

As with many medicines, initiate at a low dose and gradually titrate upwards. A gradual dose titration is particularly important to prevent potentially fatal overdose with strong opioid agonists.

Many opioids are excreted via the kidney and can accumulate in patients with renal impairment. Dosing in these patients requires particular care and dosage adjustments are commonly needed.

What are the notable adverse effects to look out for?

Mu opioid receptors mediate a number of physiological effects, and stimulation of these receptors by opioid analgesics results in both therapeutic and adverse effects. Tolerance can develop to the analgesic and some but not all of the adverse effects.

Acute administration of opioids can result in euphoria, which forms the basis of the addictive potential of these medicines. Mu receptor agonism in the brainstem results in respiratory depression, which requires careful monitoring and can be fatal.

A reduction in GI motility results in constipation (this adverse effect is utilised in the treatment of diarrhoea with loperamide) to which tolerance does not tend to develop. Certain opioids (e.g. morphine) cause rash due to histamine release, whilst nausea and vomiting are common with stronger opioids.

How can the adverse effects be minimised?

Tolerance will develop to many of the adverse effects of opioids over time. However, constipation tends to persist and may require prescription of a laxative.

The risk of dependence may be reduced by prescribing limited quantities for acute pain. Drugs used to treat nausea and vomiting may be administered if this side effect is problematic.

What needs to be monitored?

Response to treatment, respiratory rate (particularly with strong opioids), and signs of misuse.

What drug interactions are important?

Other sedative medicines (including alcohol) may cause increased drowsiness in combination with opioids. Hepatic CYP450 enzyme inducers (e.g. carbamazepine and rifampicin) may reduce the effectiveness of certain opioids.

Tramadol is a 5-hydroxytryptamine reuptake inhibitor, and combination with selective serotonin re-uptake inhibitors and other reuptake inhibitor antidepressants may result in serotonin syndrome.

Discontinuing treatment

Following longer-term treatment with full agonists, the dose should be reduced gradually prior to discontinuation to reduce the emergence of symptoms of withdrawal. Discontinuation following short-term use of weak agonists is not usually associated with withdrawal symptoms, but awareness of the possible risk and undertaking appropraite monitoring is advised.

60 Antibacterials

Commonly used antibacterial medication families and examples

Family	Examples
Aminoglycosides	Gentamycin
Carbapenems	Ertapenem
Cephalosporins	Cefuroxime
	Cefotaxime
Glycopeptide antibacterials	Teicoplanin
Lincosamides	Clindamycin
Macrolides	Clarithromycin
	Erythromycin
	Azithromycin
Monobactams	Aztreonam
Nitroimidazole derivatives	Metronidazole
Penicillins	Amoxicillin
	Phenoxymethylpenicillin
Quinolones	Ciprofloxacin
Sulphonamides	Sulfamethoxazole
Tetracyclines	Oxytetracycline
Rifamycins	Rifampicin
	Rifaximin
Miscellaneous	Chloramphenicol
	Daptomycin
	Fidaxomicin
	Fosfomycin
	Fusidic acid
	Linezolid
	Tedizolid
	Trimethoprim

Are these drugs all the same?

The medication groups listed in the table are all antibacterials (commonly referred to as 'antibiotics') and they all interfere with the bacterial life cycle. Typically, the medications interfere with the structural integrity of the bacterium (e.g. the penicillins) or with elements of reproduction of the bacteria (e.g. macrolides). The medications do not, however, have one identical common mechanism of action. They may have a broad spectrum of activity

Rapid Medicines Management for Healthcare Professionals, First Edition. Paul Deslandes, Simon Young and Ben Pitcher.
© 2020 John Wiley & Sons Ltd. Published 2020 by John Wiley & Sons Ltd.

(i.e. they will kill or reduce the reproduction of a wide range of bacterial species) or have a degree of specificity in interfering with particular bacterial subclassifications (e.g. teicoplanin has powerful activity against Gram-positive bacteria) and particular elements of their lifecycle (hence the groupings).

What are these drugs used to treat?

These medications will be used primarily to treat bacterial infections but can also be used in the prophylaxis (prevention) of infections. Antibiotics have no effect on viral infections and should not be used to treat viral illnesses such as the common cold. The use of antibacterials in the prevention of infections is reserved for particular conditions, e.g. post splenectomy and in surgical prophylaxis. The previous unwarranted use of prophylactic doses of antibiotics in healthcare has declined; the practice, if not clinically warranted, makes a significant contribution to antibiotic resistance.

What do these drugs do?

The antibacterials all interfere with the bacterium's ability to survive and/or to replicate. When a bacterium fails to replicate it cannot survive in sufficient quantity to cause clinical infection – the antibiotic action combined with the body's immune system deals with the infection.

Some of the antibacterial medications listed are *bacteriostatic* and slow the growth and reproduction of bacteria. These antibiotics will be not always be effective in those who are immunocompromised; a fully functioning immune system is required to treat an infection using bacteriostatic antibiotics. *Bactericidal* antibiotics kill bacteria; these medications are able to deal with infection even in immunocompromised patients.

What's the difference between the different types?

Penicillins and cephalosporins interfere with bacterial cell wall synthesis, which impedes bacterial growth and reproduction. Aminoglycosides and macrolides inhibit protein synthesis in the bacterial cell. Metronidazole inhibits nucleic acid synthesis by disputing the functionality of DNA in bacterial cells. Trimethoprim binds to the enzyme dihydrofolate reductase and blocks a cascade of reactions that would normally result in bacterial DNA synthesis. Quinolones like ciprofloxacin prevent the unwinding of bacterial DNA (by interfering with the topoisomerase enzyme) and thus interfere with processes such as replication and protein synthesis.

How are these drugs given?

Antibacterials are dosed by a wide variety of routes. In community-based practice most antibacterials are dosed orally in short courses ranging from 3 to 10 days dependent on the nature of the infection. The use of intravenous antibiotics is usually reserved for hard to treat infections in those who are immunocompromised, those who have co-morbidities that make them particularly vulnerable to effects of infection, and those who require an immediate effect from the antibacterial, e.g. the treatment of sepsis. Antibacterials may be administered topically, e.g. in elimination of methicillin-resistant *Staphylococcus aureus* (MRSA) prior to surgery.

Antibacterials need to be dosed regularly according to specific regimes and the course completed as prescribed unless otherwise clinically indicated. This helps prevent the development of antimicrobial resistance. Antibacterial regimes should be carefully followed. The healthcare professional should support the concordant use of these regimes for the benefit of the individual patient as well as the health of the wider population.

What are the notable adverse effects to look out for?

The adverse effects of the medications are as varied as the range of agents. Managing the adverse effects of long-term treatments is important when considering the optimisation of concordance. The *British National Formulary* and Summary of Product Characteristics detail the adverse effects of individual agents.

Diarrhoea and gastrointestinal upset are commonly reported adverse effects of antibacterials. The disruption of normal gut flora by the antibacterial often causes the diarrhoea and discomfort. The macrolides are known to be transformed into a by-product in the stomach, which causes severe gastrointestinal discomfort and diarrhoea in some patients.

Some antibiotic groups, e.g. the aminoglycosides, have particularly troublesome side effects, such as nephrotoxicity and ototoxicity, and are reserved for use when there are few alternatives. Hypersensitivity reactions are well characterised for antibiotic groups, especially the penicillins, and the role of the healthcare professional in defining the nature of the hypersensitivity response is key. Identifying true allergy from patient history is often very challenging unless the symptoms are clearly characterised. Some rashes that are described as hypersensitivity and allergy are not always true hypersensitivity responses. A thorough examination of the history of the responses is important to ensure that antibacterials are used appropriately.

What needs to be monitored?

Response to the antibacterial. Hypersensitivity reactions.

Aminoglycosides require monitoring of renal function and therapeutic drug monitoring to ensure that they are dosed optimally and to minimise the likelihood of serious adverse drug reactions.

What drug interactions are important?

Many antibiotics have been implicated in the failure of oral contraceptives. The Faculty of Sexual and Reproductive Health gives comprehensive guidance on the management of drug interactions with contraceptives. Much has been written about this topic.

https://www.fsrh.org/standards-and-guidance/documents/ceu-clinical-guidance-drug-interactions-with-hormonal.

Metronidazole interacts with alcohol. This effect can extend beyond alcohol consumed socially; liquid medicines often contain ethanol as do many cosmetic products such as aftershaves, perfumes, and deodorants. Many mouthwashes also have significant alcohol content. Each of these products can trigger an unpleasant and potentially harmful reaction with metronidazole.

Other considerations

Antimicrobial resistance is an important facet of antibacterial therapy, especially when the medications are preventing severe life-limiting infections. The importance of compliance and responsible use of antibiotics cannot be overstated.

61 Antifungals

Commonly used examples
Polyene antifungals. Amphotericin and nystatin
Triazole antifungals. Fluconazole and itraconazole
Imidazole antifungals. Miconazole and clotrimazole
Echinocandin antifungals. Caspofungin
Other. Amorolfine, griseofulvin, terbinafine

Are these drugs all the same?
The differences between different strains of fungi mean that antifungal agents can be more or less effective depending upon the organism responsible for the infection. Choice of antifungal is typically based on the location of the infection, along with the appearance of any rash or lesions. However, skin sampling for microscopy and culture can be undertaken in severe or persistent cases.

What are these drugs used to treat?
The human body can be colonised by a variety of pathological organisms. This includes yeasts and other fungi, which are most commonly associated with infections of the surface of the body, such as skin, nails or hair, or the openings into the body, such as the mouth or vagina. Nevertheless, it is possible for fungal infections to become systemic leading to sepsis.

What do these drugs do?
Antifungal agents typically work by exploiting differences between fungal and mammalian cell biology. By disrupting aspects of the fungal (but not human) cell function, they act as a poison to the fungus but not to the patient. However, this ideal is not always achievable and antifungals can cause toxicity.

What's the difference between different types?
Polyene antifungals. Amphotericin and nystatin can be used to treat a broad range of yeast and yeast-like fungi such as *Candida albicans* (thrush) and moulds such as *Aspergillus* species. Amphotericin and nystatin bind to sterols in the cell membrane, disrupting its integrity and preventing the fungus from maintaining homeostasis.
Triazole antifungals. Fluconazole and itraconazole may be used to treat or as prophylaxis against fungal infections. They inhibit the enzymes that facilitate the synthesis of ergosterols, which form the fungal cell membrane.

Rapid Medicines Management for Healthcare Professionals, First Edition. Paul Deslandes, Simon Young and Ben Pitcher.
© 2020 John Wiley & Sons Ltd. Published 2020 by John Wiley & Sons Ltd.

Imidazole antifungals. Miconazole and clotrimazole are effective against yeasts and dermatophytes (e.g. ringworm) and are even effective against some forms of bacterial infection. Like the triazole drugs, they inhibit the enzymes that facilitate the synthesis of ergosterols, which form the fungal cell membrane.

Echinocandin antifungals. These agents are only effective against specific strains of *Aspergillus* and *Candida*, inhibiting the proper formation of the fungal cell wall. They are used in the treatment of invasive or systemic infections, particularly in immunocompromised patients.

Griseofulvin is an effective choice for the treatment of certain *Trichophyton* infections such as athlete's foot and ringworm. Griseofulvin disrupts the normal mitosis in the fungal cell, preventing it from reproducing.

How are these drugs given?

Antifungals are typically given topically, directly to the site of infection. Skin, oral, or vaginal infections are usually treated using creams, solutions, or pessaries. More widespread, unresponsive, or serious infections can be treated with oral therapies or even intravenously.

Polyene antifungals. Amphotericin is given intravenously for systemic infection. Nystatin is used as an oral suspension to treat oral candidiasis and is included as an ingredient in certain creams and ointments in combination with steroids or antibacterials.

Triazole antifungals. Can be administered intravenously or orally. Fluconazole is distributed throughout the body, allowing it to be used for urinary fungal infections and even fungal meningitis.

Imidazole antifungals. These agents are used topically and can be found as creams, sprays, pessaries, and paints (to be applied to nail infections) depending on where the infection is. As creams, they are often combined with a steroid to reduce the inflammation associated with the infection.

Echinocandin antifungals. These medications are typically administered via intravenous infusion.

Griseofulvin can be administered either topically directly onto the site of infection or, if this is unsuccessful, systemically via the oral route.

Dosing

Whilst fungal infections may resolve after a short course of treatment (e.g. 7–10 days), some infections (e.g. fungal nail infections) may take many weeks or even months to resolve and require longer-term dosing.

Caution or reduced dosages are generally required in patients with renal impairment.

What are the notable adverse effects to look out for?

Polyene antifungals. Amphotericin is known to be nephrotoxic and can precipitate renal tubule damage and even acute renal failure. Administration of amphotericin can cause arrhythmias and is associated with a high incidence of allergy. Test doses should be given under close observation before the first infusion. Due to differences in the pharmacology of different preparations, amphotericin should be prescribed by brand and only the prescribed brand administered.

Triazole antifungals. This group of drugs is associated with gastrointestinal adverse effects. Fluconazole (as well as certain other triazoles) may rarely be associated with cardiac QT interval prolongation. Itraconazole is associated with liver failure and heart failure. Any indication of this in the patients should be reported at once.

Imidazole antifungals. Due to their topical application, these agents are not known to cause many adverse effects. Skin reactions may occur.

Oral use of terbinafine has been associated with liver toxicity and potentially serious skin reactions (e.g. Stevens–Johnson syndrome).

How can the adverse effects be minimised?
Prescribers may select liposomal or lipid complex amphotericin to reduce the risk of nephrotoxicity compared with conventional amphotericin-B.

What needs to be monitored?
Due to the potential for liver and renal toxicity, many antifungals require liver and renal function tests before they are commenced and throughout their use. Antifungals should be used with caution or in some cases avoided in patients with liver or renal impairment.

The triazole antifungal itraconazole may require therapeutic drug monitoring due to variations of absorption seen in conditions such as AIDS and neutropenia.

What drug interactions are important?
Many antifungal drugs are liver cytochrome enzyme inhibitors (e.g. fluconazole, miconazole) or inducers (e.g. griseofulvin). This presents a significant possibility of interactions with other drugs. The interactions appendix of the *British National Formulary* should be checked to prevent the possibility of an interaction causing patient harm.

Polyene antifungals. Whilst topical nystatin is not associated with any notable interactions, amphotericin has the potential to cause numerous severe reactions with other medications.

Triazole antifungals. These agents have many severe interactions.

Imidazole antifungals. Even though these drugs are administered topically, there is a possibility of them being absorbed and causing serious interactions with a range of drugs, including statins, coumarins, sildenafil, phenytoin, and carbamazepine. In particular, it should be noted that miconazole oral gel is swallowed and absorbed through the gastrointestinal tract and has resulted in severe harm (death) when used in combination with warfarin.

Griseofulvin has notable interactions, reducing the effectiveness of coumarins and hormonal contraceptives, increasing risk of thrombosis and unintended pregnancy, respectively.

Other considerations
Some antifungals are prescription-only medications. However, some can be bought from a pharmacy without prescription. As discussed above, miconazole has the potential for causing severe interactions with other drugs. This highlights the importance of including over-the-counter medications when checking a patient's drug history.

62 Antivirals

Commonly used antiviral families (and examples)

Medication used in the treatment of viral hepatitis. Entecavir, glecaprevir, adefovir dipivoxil, ledipasvir, peginterferon alfa, ribavirin, simeprevir, sofosbuvir.

Medication used to treat herpesvirus infections. Inosine pranobex, aciclovir, famciclovir, valaciclovir.

Medication used to treat cytomegalovirus infections. Valganciclovir, foscarnet sodium.

Medication used to treat HIV infection. Abacavir, daranuvir, dolutegravir, efavirenz, emtric-itabine, lamivudine, ritonavir, tenofovir disoproxil, zidovudine.

Medication used in the management of influenza. Oseltamivir, zanamivir.

Are these drugs all the same?

The medications/groups listed are all antivirals and they interfere with the viral lifecycle. The medications do not, however, have one common mechanism of action and they have a degree of specificity in interfering with particular viruses and particular elements of their lifecycles (hence the groupings).

What are these drugs used to treat?

The medications are typically classified as above. They are used to treat the range of viral conditions as listed.

Aciclovir, famciclovir, inosine pranobex, and valaciclovir are examples of medications used to treat cytomegalovirus and herpes species viral infections such as shingles, chicken pox, and cold sores. Oseltamivir and zanamivir reduce the replication of influenza A and B virus and are used to prevent and treat influenza. The medications used to treat HIV are dosed in combinations or regimes in order to prevent the multiplication of the HIV virus and prevent its consequent effects on the CD4 cell counts and the immune system. This prevents the development of complications associated with HIV that can cause illness and premature death. The treatment of HIV is not curative. The medications used to treat hepatitis B and C are also used as combinations and regimes to prevent the development of complications associated with these conditions.

What do these drugs do?

The antivirals all interfere with the virus' ability to replicate. When the virus fails to replicate it cannot infect tissue in the same aggressive manner and the immune system has an opportunity to fight off the viral infection. Some antiviral medications are curative and some require longer-term therapy to suppress the viral load and lessen or nullify the impact

Rapid Medicines Management for Healthcare Professionals, First Edition. Paul Deslandes, Simon Young and Ben Pitcher.

of infection. Most of the medications interfere with the enzymes that the viruses use to replicate, e.g. protease enzymes, polymerase enzymes, and neuroaminidases, and prevent the replication of the virus.

Combinations of medications are often used to increase the efficacy of the treatment but also to prevent or delay the development of resistance. Resistance is an important facet of antiviral therapy, especially when the medications are preventing severe life-limiting infections.

Ritonavir (used in the management of HIV infection) is sometimes used to 'boost' the effects of other antivirals. It achieves this as it is a potent inhibitor of cytochrome P450 enzymes and therefore reduces the metabolism of other drugs.

How are these drugs given?

Treatment of herpes virus infection and influenza. These antivirals are dosed by a variety of routes; usually orally, but also by i/v infusion or topically, where indicated.

Prevention and treatment of HIV. These antivirals are dosed primarily by mouth. Regimens typically include a combination of two or more drugs.

Treatment of viral hepatitis. The antivirals are dosed by a variety of routes, usually orally, but also via subcutaneous injection and intravenous infusion.

Dosing

All antivirals are broadly dosed in two ways. First, they are dosed in short-term courses up to several days in length to treat short-term viral infections such as shingles or to prevent influenza. The timing of commencement of antivirals can influence the duration and severity of viral illness. Second, some medications will need to be taken for many months or even for a lifetime. This is typical when attempting to treat viral conditions such as hepatitis and managing HIV.

The approach to management of hepatitis C has been changed by the introduction of drugs such as glecaprevir, ledipasvir, and sofosbuvir. These drugs are typically given in combination based on viral genotype, as a relatively short course (either 12 or 24 weeks), with the intention of curing the hepatitis C infection.

Antivirals are also dosed as pre-exposure prophylaxis (PrEP). This is an antiviral dosing regimen used when people at very high risk of being infected with HIV take medicines on a regular basis to decrease the likelihood of HIV infection. PrEP significantly reduces the risk of HIV infection in non-HIV infected individuals who may be at risk of acquiring HIV by sexual transmission and through recreational, injecting drug use.

Regimes for using antivirals constantly evolve and it is important these medications are used according to the latest evidence base. Compliance with regimes is fundamental to the most successful clinical outcomes with antivirals.

What are the notable adverse effects to look out for?

The side effects of the medications are as varied as the range of agents. Managing the adverse effects of long-term treatments is important in considering concordance. Adverse effects include (but are not limited to) hypersensitivity reactions, hyperlipidaemia, reduction in blood cell count, and psychiatric disturbance.

What needs to be monitored?

The monitoring of viral conditions is multi-faceted and consideration of alcohol consumption, sexual activity, and other aspects of social history/patient behaviour is important.

Hepatitis monitoring can include serological screening, hepatic follow-up, full blood counts, urea and electrolytes, liver function tests, thyroid function tests, HbA1c.

In treating HIV, consider full blood counts, viral load, CD4 count, medication side effects such as hypercholesterolemia and drug interactions.

The importance of compliance cannot be overstated.

What drug interactions are important?

There is a range of interactions between antivirals and other classes of drugs. The BNF has a detailed analysis of the interactions and these may be particularly clinically impactful in the case of medications use to manage hepatitis or HIV (where the efficacy of the medications needs to be sustained to maximise the clinical outcomes). In addition, deliberate appropriate polypharmacy is feature of HIV treatment, such as the use of ritonavir to enhance the effects of other antiviral drugs. It should be noted that due to its effect on cytochrome P450 enzymes, ritonavir can interact with a number of other drugs (not only antivirals).

Other considerations

The management of viral hepatitis and HIV is a specialist field and specialists initiate and have ongoing roles in managing the medications.

63 Insulin

Commonly used examples and the differences between them

Insulins are broadly divided into subtypes according to their composition, duration of action, and onset of action. Typically insulins used as medicines are divided into three types:

1. *Short-acting insulins.* These insulin types have a comparatively rapid onset of action and short duration of action (in comparison to the other two groups below). These types of insulins are often administered prior to meals (to assist with the control of the glucose associated with the meal) and used in variable rate intravenous insulin infusions for certain medical situations. Examples of short-acting insulins include Humulin S®, Actrapid®, Novorapid®, and Humalog®.
2. *Long-acting insulins.* These have a typically slower onset of action but a far longer duration of action. These are typically injected subcutaneously once or twice daily, e.g. Tresiba® (insulin degludec) and Lantus® (insulin glargine).
3. *Intermediate-acting insulins.* As the name suggests, the onset of action and duration of action are between those of the short-acting and long-acting insulin types. Examples include Humulin I® and Insulatard®.

Some insulins are available as combinations, e.g. Humulin M3 (a mixture of a short-acting and an intermediate-acting insulin in the same vial).

Insulins are typically prescribed by brand name to avoid confusion and errors relating to product selection at the point of prescribing, dispensing and administration.

Are these drugs all the same?

Although the term insulin often refers to the specific hormone present in humans and other mammals, medicinal insulins vary quite significantly (see above). Although medicinal insulin preparations are copies of the endogenous hormone, they are suitably modified to ensure their stability outside of the body and to modify their pharmacokinetic profile, which facilitates optimal blood sugar control.

What are these drugs used for?

Insulin therapy is most often used to treat type I diabetes. Patients with type I diabetes could not survive without exogenous insulin therapy. Some type II diabetics will use insulin to improve their blood glucose control when other interventions fail to adequately do so. Insulin is sometimes used in an acute setting to manage hyperkalaemia.

Rapid Medicines Management for Healthcare Professionals, First Edition. Paul Deslandes, Simon Young and Ben Pitcher.
© 2020 John Wiley & Sons Ltd. Published 2020 by John Wiley & Sons Ltd.

How do these drugs work?

Insulin is a polypeptide hormone. The hormone plays a key role in regulating the utilisation of carbohydrate, fat, and protein in the body. Insulin promotes the absorption of glucose from the blood into adipose (fat) tissue, liver, and skeletal muscle. This glucose is then converted into glycogen, fats or both (depending on the tissue). Insulin has many physiological actions over and above assisting with glucose utilisation.

In type I diabetics, where there is absolute insulin deficiency, exogenous insulin serves as a vital 'replacement' therapy for the body's inability to produce endogenous insulin. In type II diabetes insulin is used as an 'add on' therapy where there is a relative insulin deficiency and/or where resistance to the actions of insulin are present that result in poor glycaemic control.

How are these drugs given?

Insulins are given by injectable routes, primarily subcutaneously. Most patients will self-administer using a syringe and needle or by using a specific manufacturer's device, e.g. an insulin pre-filled pen. When measuring and administering insulin, if you are not using the manufacturers device *then an insulin syringe must always be used*. Insulin doses are measured in units and insulin syringes are marked so that the exact number of units will be accurately administered. Using other devices such as volumetric syringes has led to dosing errors, which can be fatal.

Dosing

Insulin doses are usually calculated using formulae dependent on the body weight of the patient. Many diabetic patients will know how to use their devices and will understand how to adjust their doses to compensate for increased food consumption, changes in exercise regimes etc. Certain circumstances, e.g. infection, trauma, and certain co-morbidities, may alter typical insulin requirements.

Insulin is usually administered as a 'regime'. Examples include the basal–bolus regime in which a basal (long-acting/intermediate-acting) insulin is usually administered once or twice daily and bolus doses of rapid/short-acting insulin are administered typically three times daily (e.g. just before or after meals). This is a fairly flexible regime but requires somewhere between three and five injections per day dependent on the patient's insulin type and their pattern of food consumption (and other lifestyle factors that affect glucose control). Other regimens also used include fixed-dose therapies, flexible therapies, insulin pump therapy, and sliding scales (variable rate).

What are the notable adverse effects to look out for?

The most common side effects associated with insulin therapy are hypoglycaemia and lipodystrophy (a lump in the skin associated with fat accumulation at the insulin injection site).

How can the adverse effects be minimised?

Hypoglycaemia is a sign of insulin overdose and needs to be carefully monitored regardless of the circumstances and the setting of care. Lipodystrophy is best prevented by the rotation of injection sites.

What needs to be monitored?

Diabetic patients should be offered a range of biopsychosocial support and health monitoring because poor diabetic control can lead to complications that, in the long term, are potentially more challenging than the acute problems associated with diabetes.

Patients treated with insulin will undertake routine monitoring of blood glucose levels. Targets are set to avoid hypoglycaemia and optimise blood glucose control; hypoglycaemia and driving are a particular issue to take into account. Monitoring will continue if the patient moves between healthcare settings. Care should be taken to ensure that blood glucose is checked prior to administration, particularly in an inpatient setting.

The HbA1c level is a blood test that provides a measure of how well-controlled blood glucose has been in previous months. HbA1c is typically measured every three to six months. The target range of HbA1c for a type I diabetic is 48 mmol mol^{-1} (6.5%) or lower. The better controlled the HbA1c the less significant the risk of development of diabetes-related complications.

What drug interactions are important?

There are few clinically significant drug interactions with insulin; most interactions relate to enhancement or interference with glycaemic control.

Other considerations

- Insulin is stored in the refrigerator prior to use. Show the vial to the patient prior to administration.
- Care should be taken as insulin dosages are measured in units and should be prescribed as such.
- Tresiba is available as 100 and 200 units per ml – care.

64 Blood Glucose Lowering Drugs

Commonly used examples

Acarbose.

Dipeptidyl peptidase-4 (DPP-4) inhibitors, e.g. alogliptin, linagliptin, saxagliptin, sitagliptin, and vildagliptin.

Glucagon-like peptide-1 (GLP-1) receptor agonists, e.g. albiglutide, dulaglutide, exenatide, liraglutide, and lixisenatide.

Meglitinides, e.g. nateglinide and repaglinide.

Metformin (a biguanide).

Pioglitazone (a thiazolidinedione).

Sodium-glucose co-transporter-2 (SGLT-2) inhibitors, e.g. canagliflozin, dapagliflozin, and empagliflozin.

Sulfonylureas, e.g. gliclazide and glipizide.

Are these drugs all the same?

The antiglycaemic medications listed above all have the same broad pharmacodynamic aim of lowering blood glucose. However, the mechanisms by which they do so and routes of administration are different (see below).

What are these drugs used to treat?

This group of medications is mainly used for the treatment of type II diabetes. Their function is primarily the reduction of blood glucose with the aim of reducing the risk of the micro- and macrovascular complications of type II diabetes. As can be seen from their mechanisms of action, many of these drugs need a pancreas that is capable of insulin secretion, so have no value in blood glucose management in type I diabetes. Metformin is also used to treat polycystic ovarian syndrome (PCOS).

What do these drugs do?

Type II diabetes is an endocrine disorder characterised by an inability of the body to appropriately metabolise glucose. Features of type II diabetes include deviations from normal insulin production and secretion, beta cell dysfunction and decreased insulin sensitivity; the net result is hyperglycaemia. This can be treated by lifestyle modification and/or medication; this group of medications is used to lower blood sugars.

Acarbose inhibits an enzyme group in the gastrointestinal (GI) tract (alpha-glucosidases) and delays the absorption of starch and sucrose. The medication also causes a delay in digestion of starch and sucrose. This causes a lowering of post-prandial (after a meal) blood glucose elevation.

Rapid Medicines Management for Healthcare Professionals, First Edition. Paul Deslandes, Simon Young and Ben Pitcher.
© 2020 John Wiley & Sons Ltd. Published 2020 by John Wiley & Sons Ltd.

Incretin hormones, such as GLP-1, are released by the GI tract throughout the day and secretion increases in response to consumption of a meal. Hormones like GLP-1 cause an increase in the release of insulin and improve glucose homeostasis. The *GLP-1 receptor agonists* mimic the effects of the incretins at their receptor sites. The *DPP-4 inhibitors* inhibit DPP-4 (an enzyme responsible for the breakdown of incretins) and prolong and sustain the action of endogenous incretins, especially GLP-1.

The *meglitinides* are usually taken prior to meals and control the 'spike' in blood glucose caused by the meal. They produce this effect by stimulating the production of insulin.

Metformin activates a liver enzyme that results in an increase in the sensitivity of cells to insulin, increases glucose utilisation, and inhibits gluconeogenesis (the production of glucose endogenously). *Pioglitazone* enhances the expression of certain genes in cells. The net effect is reduced insulin resistance, improved cellular utilisation of glucose, and reduced blood glucose.

The *SGLT-2 inhibitors* block a pathway that prevents the resorption of glucose from urine in the kidney. In non-diabetic individuals glucose is not found in urine. The body utilises a transporter protein to resorb the glucose as urine is formed. If this transport protein is blocked by SGLT-2 inhibitors, glucose will be excreted in urine. In diabetics, this is a useful mechanism for removing excess glucose from urine (and hence lowering blood sugar). As a result, they may lead to some weight loss, and also have a mild diuretic effect, which can help to reduce blood pressure.

The *sulfonylureas* bind to channels in the beta cells of the pancreas and trigger the release of insulin from those beta cells (the sulfonylureas are often termed insulin secretagogues as they stimulate the secretion of insulin).

How are these drugs given?

All of the medications are given by mouth with the exception of the GLP-1 receptor agonists. The GLP-1 receptor agonists are polypeptides and are administered by subcutaneous injection.

In addition to these drug groups, type II diabetics may take medication to manage their blood pressure and lipid profile, and prevent cardiovascular events. This is a classical case of *appropriate polypharmacy*.

Dosing

All of these medications are taken regularly using fixed regimes or are titrated upwards to achieve the desired blood glucose level. Initial treatment is typically with metformin monotherapy, although many patients will take more than one of these medications to improve glycaemic control. There are some specific licenced combination products of the drugs such as Janumet® (a tablet containing a fixed dose of both metformin and sitagliptin), which may help with treatment adherence. Some drugs are available as both immediate-release and sustained-release products, which are not interchangeable, as the differing pharmacokinetic profiles will require differing dosing regimens to produce the desired clinical effect.

As with many medicines, hepatic and renal function is important in the metabolism and elimination of certain antiglycaemics. Impairment in the functioning of these organs may require dosage alterations or avoidance of specific drugs (e.g. SGLT-2 inhibitors when estimated glomerular filtration rate [eGFR] is reduced).

What are the notable adverse effects to look out for?

The adverse effect that causes most concern with certain antiglycaemics is hypoglycaemia. Hypoglycaemia is a problematic side effect, especially when considered in the context of driving and operating heavy machinery. The degree of hypoglycaemia varies according to the type of antiglycaemic medicine. Weight gain can also be problematic with certain types of antiglycaemic.

Acarbose can cause flatulence and abdominal discomfort. DPP-4 inhibitors also cause abdominal pain and GI upset, and are associated with a small risk of pancreatitis. GLP-1 agonists also cause abdominal discomfort and there are also warnings about the possible development of pancreatitis. The meglitinides have few side effects of note, barring hypersensitivity reactions. Metformin commonly causes GI upset. More rarely it can be associated with lactic acidosis, a serious adverse effect that may be more common when renal function is impaired. Metformin does not typically cause weight gain and when used alone does not cause hypoglycaemia.

The SGLT-2 inhibitors have been associated with the development of euglycaemic diabetic ketoacidosis (DKA). Due to increased levels of glucose in the urine, as part of their mechanism of action, these drugs may also increase the risk of urinary tract infections. The sulphonylureas can cause hypoglycaemia, although this is uncommon and occurs at higher doses. They also tend to cause weight gain. Pioglitazone has warnings relating to cardiovascular safety (heart failure) and bladder cancer, and may commonly cause weight gain.

How can the adverse effects be minimised?

Adverse effects can be minimised by appropriate monitoring of blood sugars and known adverse effects. Switching between different drug types may be required to find a drug that is tolerated best by an individual patient.

What needs to be monitored?

Blood glucose, HbA1c, urine testing (for ketones and glucose), renal function, and monitoring for diabetes and its associated complications.

What drug interactions are important?

There are few severe drug interactions associated with antiglycaemic agents. Metabolism via hepatic cytochrome P450 enzymes occurs with some of the drugs, and they may interact with the inducers or inhibitors of these enzymes.

Other considerations

The use of this group of medications is increasing as the incidence of type II diabetes increases. There is specific advice from the manufacturers with regard to the use of these medications in pregnancy and breast-feeding, and for appropriate use prior to surgical intervention.

65 Steroids

The term steroids is often used to describe corticosteroids and this chapter will focus on these treatments. However, oestrogens and progestogens found in oral contraceptives, hormone replacement therapy, and the anabolic steroids often misused as performance-enhancing drugs (PEDs) by athletes are also steroidal in nature but have differing indications and side-effect profiles from the steroid examples listed below.

Commonly used examples

Glucocorticoid: betamethasone, dexamethasone, fluticasone, mometasone, prednisolone.
  Mineralocorticoid: fludrocortisone.
  Mixed glucocorticoid and mineralocorticoid: hydrocortisone.

Are these drugs all the same?

Corticosteroids are hormones produced by the adrenal gland (specifically the adrenal cortex). There are two main categories/pharmacological groups: the glucocorticoids and the mineralocorticoids. As well as the naturally occurring steroids there are synthetic analogues that are used medicinally (see Table 65.1).

What are these drugs used for?

The steroids have a wide variety of uses medicinally. Glucocorticoids such as dexamethasone reduce inflammation, as well as having effects on metabolism, including influencing the metabolism of carbohydrates and fats. Mineralocorticoids such as aldosterone and fludrocortisone influence water and electrolyte homeostasis by affecting the transport of ions in the kidney. Overall, steroids are utilised to a greater extent for their anti-inflammatory and immunosuppressive properties. The steroids with glucocorticoid activity have important roles in influencing the course of immune and inflammatory responses in conditions such as asthma, eczema, multiple sclerosis, and some cancer chemotherapy regimens. Dexamethasone is used in a range of conditions, e.g. in the management of croup, to stimulate appetite in anorexia, and to reduce cerebral oedema associated with malignancies (see Table 65.2).

What's the difference between different types?

There is a wide range of steroids used medicinally. Each steroid has its own set of features and properties that make it most suitable for a given formulation and indication. Some steroids, such as clobetasol, are primarily applied topically and are not suitable for oral or systemic use. Steroids like hydrocortisone are used for a wider range of conditions and are administered through a wider range of formulations.

Rapid Medicines Management for Healthcare Professionals, First Edition. Paul Deslandes, Simon Young and Ben Pitcher.
© 2020 John Wiley & Sons Ltd. Published 2020 by John Wiley & Sons Ltd.

Table 65.1 Examples of endogenous and synthetic steroids important in physiology and medicine.

Endogenous steroid	Exogenous analogue	Synthetic analogue
Cortisol	Hydrocortisone	Prednisolone
Aldosterone	—	Fludrocortisone

Table 65.2 Examples of commonly used steroids, their indications, and routes of administration.

Steroid	Indication	Formulation/route of administration
Betamethasone	Eye inflammation	Eye drop/ointment
Budesonide	Asthma	Inhalation of powder
Clobetasol	Eczema	Cream/ointment
Fluticasone	Asthma	Inhalation of aerosol (pressurised device/nebulisation)
Hydrocortisone/fludrocortisone	Addison's disease	Orally (tablets)
Methylprednisolone	Treatment of relapse in multiple sclerosis	Injection
Prednisolone	Asthma	Orally (tablets)
Prednisolone	Ulcerative colitis	Foam enema

How do these drugs work?

Both glucocorticoids and mineralocorticoids bind to receptor subtypes in the cytosol to form a complex. This complex becomes activated then crosses the nuclear membrane, where it binds to specific targets in the DNA. This regulates gene transcription and influences the behaviour of the cell type affected. This process is known as transactivation. In addition, other processes can occur, such as transpression, where the complex binds to another region of DNA and suppresses transcription. Some of the anti-inflammatory actions of steroids are due to the transactivation of anti-inflammatory genes and the suppression of pro-inflammatory genes. Steroids also have non-genomic effects: they influence targets such as signalling cascades that do not involve nuclear targets.

How are these drugs given?

Steroids are administered or taken in a wide variety of ways. Patients with Addison's disease take regular oral steroids to replace the endogenous cortisol that the body is unable to produce. If the steroid is being administered to treat inflammation in a particular region of the body, a route of administration may be used to act more directly on that area and reduce the systemic effect. Asthma patients may take regular inhaled corticosteroids and in addition may require short courses (usually a number of days) of oral steroids should their condition worsen. Eczema patients may use topical steroids regularly for short periods of time to deal with flare-ups of their condition. Patients with inflammatory bowel disease may use enemas or rectal foams for short periods to deliver drugs to the lower intestine and manage flare-ups of their condition.

Dosing

The introduction of steroids to a patient's medication regime will depend on the purpose of the steroid and its role in influencing the disease process. Many short courses do not require titration, e.g. steroids such as oral prednisolone may be initiated at a dose of 40 mg daily (usually in the morning) for five days without up-titration or a slow down-titration when the course is complete. In the case of polymyalgia rheumatica, the condition often needs treating with steroids for months or years. Steroid eye drops used post-operatively will often be used until the inflammation associated with the procedure has subsided. Doses of dexamethasone for croup can be single doses in mild cases or typically three doses in more severe cases (subject to review).

What are the notable adverse effects to look out for?

Systemic. Bruising, Cushing's syndrome, menstrual irregularities, increased appetite (weight gain), increased susceptibility to infection (e.g. chickenpox), more severe responses to infection, insomnia, growth suppression (in children), psychiatric reactions (e.g. mood changes) and water retention. Steroids given orally can cause gastric irritation.

Topical. Potent steroids administered topically can be absorbed through the skin and may be associated with systemic adverse effects.

How can the adverse effects be minimised?

Primarily by using the minimum effective dose for the shortest possible duration. Formulations allowing drug delivery to the specific tissue to be treated (e.g. skin, lung, joint) will help to reduce absorption into the circulation and reduce systemic adverse effects.

What drug interactions are important?

Corticosteroids will antagonise the hypotensive effects of antihypertensive drugs such as beta-blockers, angiotensin converting enzyme inhibitors, and alpha-blockers.

Steroids interact with a number of drugs used to treat epilepsy, e.g. carbamazepine (enzyme induction by the carbamazepine increases the metabolism of the steroid). Steroids can enhance or reduce the effect of warfarin and the coumarins. High doses of steroids should not be used with live vaccines.

Discontinuing treatment

Patients may carry a steroid card (especially in longer-term use) warning that abrupt withdrawal of treatment is inappropriate. During long periods of systemic steroid use, the adrenal glands can atrophy and stop producing endogenous steroids. This suppression may persist for many years and abrupt discontinuation of steroid treatment can cause severe illness or even death. Adjustments to steroid doses may need to be made, e.g. during intercurrent illness, trauma, and surgical procedures, to avoid significant falls in blood pressure. Abrupt discontinuation may precipitate a worsening of the condition that the steroid is treating.

Long-term systemic steroid use requires a carefully considered withdrawal regime to a minimum effective dose or complete discontinuation. The parameters for the requirement to manage a steroid withdrawal are found in guidelines and the rate of discontinuation is often considered on a clinical case-by-case basis.

66 Contraceptives

There is a variety of contraceptive methods available. This section focuses on hormonal contraception and its medicines management considerations. Hormonal methods are evidenced to be the most reliable forms of contraception. Oral contraceptives are sometimes called 'the pill', combined hormonal/oral contraceptives, or progestogen-only pill (POP).

Commonly used examples
Hormonal contraceptives broadly fall into four categories:

1. *Combined hormonal contraceptives (sometimes known as combined oral contraceptives).* Cilest®, Marvelon®, Mercilon®, and Yasmin®.
2. *Oral progestogen-only contraceptives.* Cerazette®, Cerelle®, Noriday®, and Primolut N®.
3. *Emergency hormonal contraception.* Levonelle One Step®.
4. *Parenteral progestogen-only contraception.* Nexplanon® (implant), and Depo-Provera® (intramuscular injection).

Intrauterine systems impregnated with hormones are also available, e.g. the Mirena® intrauterine device.

Are these drugs all the same?
Each of the categories above offers an appropriate, efficacious level of contraception. The selection of a method should be patient-centred with consideration that there are, as with all medications, risks with using certain products across the spectrum of women who may choose to use the methods. Some of the medications are licenced for use for menstrual disorders such as dysmenorrhea and menorrhagia as well as for contraceptive purposes.

What's the difference between different types?
Combined hormonal contraceptives
The combined hormonal contraceptives (CHCs) contain a combination of two analogues of the female sex hormones (oestrogen and progesterone). The most commonly used oestrogen analogue is ethinylestradiol but estradiol and mestranol can be also be found in CHCs. Examples of the progestogens found in CHCs include desogestrel, gestodene, and levonorgestrel. The CHCs are classified into low and standard strength preparations. The low strength CHCs are usually used for women who exhibit certain risk factors for circulatory disease (and where the CHC is otherwise indicated).

These medications are generally indicated for contraceptive purposes and the management of menstrual disorders.

Rapid Medicines Management for Healthcare Professionals, First Edition. Paul Deslandes, Simon Young and Ben Pitcher.
© 2020 John Wiley & Sons Ltd. Published 2020 by John Wiley & Sons Ltd.

There is a significant list of cautions and contraindications associated with CHC use. Contraindications include history of breast cancer, migraine with aura, and personal history of arterial disease. Risk factors that form part of a key decision as to whether CHCs are suitable for a woman include (but are not limited to) family history of thromboembolic disease, obesity, long-term immobility, smoking, and age (>35 years).

Oral progestogen-only contraceptives

These pills contain analogues of progesterone known as progestogens. They contain no oestrogen analogues. These medications are generally indicated for contraceptive purposes and the management of menstrual disorders. They have a number of contraindications and cautions but they are available to a broader group of women than the CHCs.

Emergency hormonal contraception

These pills contain analogues of progesterone known as progestogens. The dose of progestogens in these tablets is significantly higher than the dose found in oral progestogen-only contraceptives.

They are indicated for emergency contraception (see dosing below) and have similar cautions and contraindications to oral progestogen-only contraceptives.

Parenteral progestogen-only contraception

These formulations contain analogues of progesterone known as progestogens. They are injectable formulations and have durations of action ranging from months to years depending on which formulation is used. They are generally indicated for contraceptive purposes and the management of menstrual disorders.

How do these drugs work?

The hormones act to prevent pregnancy by altering sex hormone homeostasis. This leads to a multiple mode of action centred on preventing ovulation, thinning the uterine lining, and thickening the mucous produced by the cervix. All of these actions are not conducive to implantation and sustaining a pregnancy.

How are these drugs given and dosed?
Combined hormonal contraceptives

There are three presentations of these pills depending on the brand. *The manufacturers' instructions need to be followed.*

1. *Monophasic pill – 28 day cycle.* The patient takes active CHC pills for 21 days (each pill contains an identical amount of the two hormones) then has a seven-day break, e.g. Yasmin®.
2. *Everyday pill (ED) – 28 day cycle (21 + 7).* The patient take active CHC pills for 21 days (each pill contains an identical amount of the two hormones) then takes seven days of placebo pill containing no hormones, e.g. Microgynon ED®.
3. *Phasic pill – 28 day cycle.* These formulations have two or three different pills in a pack that contain varying amounts of hormone and need to be taken in the correct order for 21 days. There is a break of seven days at the end of the cycle, e.g. Logynon®.

Oral progestogen-only contraceptives

Oral progestogen-only contraceptives are taken once a day at approximately the same time each day on an ongoing basis.

Emergency hormonal contraception

These formulations are taken as a single dose. They need to be taken within a fixed time frame after unprotected sex. These medications are available from pharmacies as well as clinics and GPs.

Parenteral progestogen-only contraception

These are injected or implanted as per the manufacturer's instructions.

What are the notable adverse effects to look out for?

These vary across the contraceptive types but include nausea, vomiting, breast tenderness, headache, and menstrual irregularities. There are warnings around the long-term effects of the use of these medications. CHCs are associated with an increased risk of cardiovascular adverse effects and this is a factor in treatment choice.

What needs to be monitored?

Regular appointments must be kept to ensure the ongoing well-being of the woman and a review of the efficacy and suitability of the medication undertaken. Advice should be sought regarding what actions need to be taken if vomiting or diarrhoea occur or if the woman falls pregnant whilst taking using the contraceptive.

What drug interactions are important?

Contraceptives interact with a range of medicines. Those that have the most impact are the interactions between the oral contraceptives and antibiotics, and oral contraceptives with anti-epileptics due to the risk of treatment failure.

Other considerations

In order to sustain contraceptive efficacy these contraceptives need to be started at particular times of the menstrual cycle or additional precautions need to be taken until the efficacy of the contraceptive is established. There are rules that govern the management of missed pills; time limits exist for each product in order to maintain efficacy if pills are missed. The BNF provides general advice but the summary of product characteristics will provide more detail for a given product.

67 Drugs for Urinary Incontinence and Retention

Commonly used examples

Urinary incontinence

Antimuscarinic drugs (sometimes referred to as anticholinergic drugs), e.g. oxybutynin, solifenacin, tolterodine, trospium.

Serotonin and noradrenaline reuptake inhibitors (SNRIs), e.g. duloxetine (see Chapter 50).

Urinary retention

Alpha-receptor antagonists, e.g. alfuzosin, doxazosin, indoramin, prazosin, tamsulosin.

5α-reductase inhibitors, e.g. dutasteride, finasteride.

Are these drugs all the same?

Drugs used for urinary incontinence and urinary retention are usually divided into different groups according to their mechanism of action. Drugs from the same group typically have similar pharmacodynamic properties, but drugs from different groups may vary significantly.

What are these drugs used to treat?

Drugs for urinary incontinence help to reduce nocturnal enuresis, as well as urinary incontinence and frequency. The SNRI duloxetine is also licensed as an antidepressant.

Drugs for urinary retention help to facilitate the passage of urine and are typically used for men with benign prostatic hypertrophy (enlargement), which is associated with a physiological impairment to the flow of urine. The alpha-blocking group of drugs are sometimes used in the treatment of certain cardiovascular conditions.

What do these drugs do?

Antimuscarinic drugs

Stimulation of detrusor muscles in the bladder by the parasympathetic nervous system results in contraction of the bladder and urination. Antimuscarinic drugs inhibit the effects of the parasympathetic nervous system by blocking the muscarinic acetylcholine receptors responsible for stimulation of bladder smooth muscle. Muscarinic receptors are also found in many other body tissues and organs, and the action of the drugs at these sites may result in adverse effects. Some members of this group (e.g. solifenacin) are more selective for the M_3 muscarinic receptor, which may help to reduce adverse effects mediated through other muscarinic receptor subtypes.

Rapid Medicines Management for Healthcare Professionals, First Edition. Paul Deslandes, Simon Young and Ben Pitcher.
© 2020 John Wiley & Sons Ltd. Published 2020 by John Wiley & Sons Ltd.

Drugs for urinary retention

Alpha-receptor antagonists. Contraction of prostate smooth muscle is mediated by the action of the sympathetic nervous system acting on adrenergic alpha$_1$-receptors. This contraction inhibits the normal flow of urine. Alpha-receptor antagonists block the action of the sympathetic nervous system, facilitating prostate smooth muscle relaxation and urinary flow.

5α-reductase inhibitors. Prostate gland enlargement causes pressure on the urethra, inhibiting the flow of urine. Prostate enlargement is mediated by the action of dihydrotestosterone, a metabolite of testosterone. Conversion of testosterone to dihydrotestosterone is facilitated by the enzyme 5α-reductase. By inhibiting the action of this enzyme, 5α-reductase inhibitors, such as finasteride, help to reduce prostate enlargement and increase urinary flow.

What's the difference between different types?

Drugs for urinary incontinence and urinary frequency have opposing effects. The former help to reduce the flow of urine, whilst the latter help to facilitate it.

Drugs for urinary incontinence aim to stabilise the muscles responsible for bladder emptying, reducing symptoms of urgency and increasing bladder capacity.

Drugs used to treat urinary retention caused by prostate hypertrophy either increase smooth muscle relaxation or help to attenuate the enlargement of the prostate gland to facilitate the flow of urine.

How are these drugs given?

Regularly, by mouth, as tablets or capsules. Regular review of the need for ongoing treatment is required.

Dosing

Some of the antimuscarinic drugs are short acting and must be given several times a day, whilst others are longer acting, allowing once daily dosing.

Alpha-receptor antagonists are typically given once or twice a day. Tamsulosin has a relatively short half-life and is formulated as a modified-release preparation to allow once-daily dosing.

5α-reductase inhibitors are given once a day.

What are the notable adverse effects to look out for?

Antimuscarinic effects such as blurred vision, dry mouth, constipation, sedation, and confusion result from muscarinic acetylcholine receptor antagonism in different parts of the body. Confusion in elderly patients is a particular concern (see the other considerations section).

Alpha-receptor antagonists are sometimes used in the management of hypertension and may cause postural hypotension and palpitations.

5α-reductase inhibitors may cause decreased libido and sexual dysfunction. More rarely, they have been associated with depression and suicidal ideation. These drugs are teratogenic and cause congenital abnormalities in the male foetus.

How can the adverse effects be minimised?

Antimuscarinics. Many drugs from diverse groups (e.g. antidepressants, antipsychotics, antihistamines) have antimuscarinic effects. Avoiding using combinations of these drugs is important to minimise additive antimuscarinic effects, particularly confusion in elderly patients.

Alpha-receptor antagonists. Doses of certain examples are increased gradually to help improve tolerability.

5α-reductase inhibitors. Women of child-bearing potential should take care not to handle broken tablet or capsule formulations of dutasteride or finasteride to minimise any risk of congenital abnormality. Effective contraception is required to avoid exposure of female partners of child-bearing potential to these drugs.

What needs to be monitored?

Treatment outcome and the need for ongoing therapy should be reviewed on a regular basis.

What drug interactions are important?

Antimuscarinics. As mentioned above, the use of combinations of drugs with antimuscarinic properties should be minimised where possible, particularly in the elderly. Inhibitors of cytochrome P450 enzymes such as macrolide antibacterials (e.g. clarithromycin) and antifungals (e.g. itraconazole and ketoconazole) can increase plasma levels of certain antimuscarinics.

Alpha-receptor antagonists. Use of alpha-receptor antagonists in combination with other antihypertensives will result in an increased hypotensive effect.

5α-reductase inhibitors. No clinically significant interactions have currently been identified.

Discontinuing treatment

For all of these medications, discontinuation of treatment may result in a return of symptoms. Patients should consult their prescriber before considering discontinuation.

Other considerations

Anticholinergic burden and its impact on cognition and memory are a concern, particularly in elderly patients. Several resources are available that outline the relative anticholinergic effects of a range of different drugs. These can be used to help minimise exposure to combinations of drugs with anticholinergic properties.

The handling of 5α-reductase inhibitors by women of child-bearing potential involved in drug administration requires particular care and caution.

68 Drugs for Osteoporosis

Commonly used examples

Bisphosphonates, e.g. alendronic acid and risedronate sodium.
   Calcium and vitamin D supplements, e.g. calcitriol.
   Raloxifene, denosumab, teriparatide.

What are these drugs used to treat?

Bisphosphonates. Postmenopausal osteoporosis, osteoporosis in men and in the prevention
      and treatment of corticosteroid-induced osteoporosis. Risedronate is also indicated
      for the treatment of Paget's disease of bone.

Calcium and vitamin D supplements. Prevention and treatment of calcium and vitamin D
      deficiency.

Raloxifene. Treatment and prevention of postmenopausal osteoporosis.

Denosumab. Osteoporosis in postmenopausal women and in men at increased risk of frac-
      tures, bone loss associated with hormone ablation in men with prostate cancer at
      increased risk of fractures. Bone loss associated with long-term systemic glucocorti-
      coid therapy in patients at increased risk of fracture.

Teriparatide. Treatment of osteoporosis in post-menopausal women and in men at increased
      risk of fractures and the treatment of corticosteroid induced osteoporosis.

What do these drugs do?

In osteoporosis, the normal homeostasis of bone reconstruction and bone resorption (loss)
tips in favour of bone loss. This does not change the appearance of bone but the structure
and strength of bone is affected, leaving the patient more prone to fractures. This is typically most important in post-menopausal women and elderly patients. The medication used
to treat osteoporosis aims to redress the balance back in favour of bone reconstruction, to
try to prevent or reduce the impact of bone resorption and reduce the incidence of the
consequences such as fractures.

What's the difference between different types?

The medications used to treat osteoporosis are all quite different. In order for some of the
groups to work effectively, many (e.g. alendronic acid) will be prescribed alongside calcium
and vitamin D supplements. Adequate blood levels of calcium and vitamin D must be maintained in order to prevent and treat osteoporosis. The bisphosphonates inhibit the bone
resorption process. Vitamin D is necessary for the absorption and utilisation of calcium.
Calcium is important in the formation of bone tissue (and a range of other biochemical
processes). Raloxifene is an oestrogen receptor modulator and is used in the prevention and

Rapid Medicines Management for Healthcare Professionals, First Edition. Paul Deslandes,
Simon Young and Ben Pitcher.
© 2020 John Wiley & Sons Ltd. Published 2020 by John Wiley & Sons Ltd.

treatment of osteoporosis. Denosumab binds with high affinity to receptor activator of nuclear factor Kappa-B ligand (RANKL), preventing the activation of receptor activator of nuclear factor Kappa-B (RANK) and thus inhibiting osteoclast formation and thus bone resorption. Teriparatide mimics the effect of parathyroid hormone and stimulates the formation of bone by exerting a direct effect on osteoblasts (the cells that promote the formation of bone).

Dosing

Bisphosphonates. Alendronic acid is given regularly, orally (tablet, effervescent tablet, and oral solution). The usual dosing is 10 mg daily or 70 mg once weekly. Risedronate sodium is dosed at 5 mg daily or 35 mg weekly for osteoporosis.

Calcium and vitamin D supplements are dosed orally. There is a range of products available and the dosing is undertaken in accordance with the degree of deficiency.

Raloxifene. Orally at 60 mg a day on a regular basis.

Denosumab (Prolia) is dosed as a single subcutaneous injection once every six months into the thigh, abdomen, or upper arm.

Teriparatide is a subcutaneous injectable product that is dosed at 20 micrograms daily. There is a maximum duration of treatment of 24 months and the course of treatment is not to be repeated.

How are these drugs given?

Alendronic acid and risedronate sodium formulations should be swallowed whole and not chewed or broken, soon after the patient gets up in morning. The oral solution (alendronic acid) should be swallowed in one single dose. Each dose should be taken with plenty of water while the patient is sitting or standing and the patient needs to remain standing or sitting upright for 30 minutes after dosing. Alendronic acid formulations should be taken on an empty stomach or at least 30 minutes before a meal or other medication. In the case of risedronate sodium formulations, food (especially calcium-containing products, e.g. dairy products) and some mineral supplements interfere with the action of the medication; they should be avoided two hours before or after risedronate consumption.

Calcium and vitamin D supplements are often available as chewable tablets and some are physically quite large dosage forms.

What are the notable adverse effects to look out for?

Bisphosphonates. Gastrointestinal side effects such as bloating and dyspepsia. Oesophageal symptoms such as pain on swallowing or dysphagia ✤. Other more rare side effects include eye disorders and osteonecrosis of the jaw.

Calcium and vitamin D. Gastrointestinal side effects and disorders of calcium homeostasis.

Raloxifene. Hot flushes (and other vascular effects) and leg cramps.

Denosumab. Associated with a risk of osteonecrosis of the jaw and with a risk of hypocalcaemia.

Teriparatide. Gastrointestinal disorders, muscle cramps, sweating.

What needs to be monitored?

This will depend upon the specific medicine, but commonly:

blood calcium levels
parathyroid blood tests
scans to assess bone density and monitor the progress of the condition
medication side effects.

What drug interactions are important?

Bisphosphonates. The interaction with foods is probably most significant. If patients are taking non-steroidal anti-inflammatory drugs then gastrointestinal and oesophageal side effects may become an important feature to monitor.

Calcium salts. Thiazide diuretics reduce urinary excretion of calcium and may increase the risk of hypercalcaemia. Calcium salts interact with tetracyclines (reduced tetracycline absorption) and can interfere with absorption of bisphosphonates (see dosing of bis-phosphonates above); quinolone antibiotic absorption can be affected by calcium salts.

Other considerations

The strength of vitamin D is measured in international units (units) not in milligrams or micrograms. The units are a measure of biological activity because vitamin D is not one single substance, but a mixture of related compounds.

69 Vitamins

Vitamins are essential nutrients that are needed by the body to allow normal physiological functioning. They are involved with a wide range of processes and deficiency can be associated with different disease states.

Commonly used examples

Vitamin name	Chemical name (examples of brand(s) encountered)	Indications	Physiological function(s)	Fat or water soluble/notes
A	Retinol (unavailable as a single-ingredient preparation; part of multivitamin preparations)	Prevention and treatment of deficiency Retinoid derivatives (e.g. isotretinoin) are used in the treatment of severe acne	Supports immune and ocular function (deficiency rare in the UK)	[a]Often found combined with other fat-soluble vitamins in multivitamin preparations Antioxidant
D	Alfacalcidol, colecalciferol, ergocalciferol (One-alpha®, Fultium D$_3$®)	Prevention and treatment of vitamin D and calcium deficiency (especially in renal disease and osteoporosis)	Renal function and utilised to ensure appropriate absorption of calcium and phosphate (important in bone health)	[a]Often contained in medications containing calcium Exists as many analogues Deficiency leads to rickets and can occur in patients who do not receive sufficient sunlight
E	Tocopherol (non-proprietary)	Prevention and treatment of deficiency	Involved in nerve conduction and in the prevention of anaemia	[a]
K	Menadiol sodium phosphate and phytomenadione (Konakion®)	Prevention and treatment of deficiency Reversal of anticoagulation with warfarin/prior to surgery (if indicated)	Required for correct functioning of the clotting cascade	[a]Konakion MM paediatric® injection is sometimes given by mouth if oral administration is required

(Continued)

Rapid Medicines Management for Healthcare Professionals, First Edition. Paul Deslandes, Simon Young and Ben Pitcher.
© 2020 John Wiley & Sons Ltd. Published 2020 by John Wiley & Sons Ltd.

Vitamin name	Chemical name (examples of brand(s) encountered)	Indications	Physiological function(s)	Fat or water soluble/notes
B$_1$	Thiamine (Pabrinex® along with other water-soluble vitamins)	Prevention and treatment of deficiency Important in the management of Wernicke – Korsakoff syndrome and its prevention	Co-enzyme used in the generation of energy in the cell	[b]Serious allergic reactions have occurred after parenteral use The MHRA have produced guidance on its prevention and management
B$_2$	Riboflavin (unavailable as a single-ingredient preparation; part of multivitamin preparations)	Prevention and treatment of deficiency Ariboflavinosis is rare in the west	Co-enzyme used in metabolic processes	[b]
B$_3$	Niacin (unavailable as a single-ingredient preparation; part of multivitamin preparations)	Prevention and treatment of deficiency	Co-enzyme used in metabolic processes and lipid metabolism	[b]
B$_5$	Pantothenic acid (unavailable as a single-ingredient preparation; part of multivitamin preparations)	Prevention and treatment of deficiency	Co-enzyme used in metabolic processes	[b]
B$_6$	Pyridoxine (non-proprietary)	Prevention and treatment of deficiency Treatment of iatrogenic neuropathy	Co-enzyme used in metabolic processes and supports red blood cell formation	[b]Deficiency can rarely occur following isoniazid or penicillamine use
B$_7$	Biotin (unavailable as a single-ingredient preparation; part of multivitamin preparations)	Prevention and treatment of deficiency	Co-enzyme used in metabolic processes	[b]
B$_9$	Folic acid (many brands/non-proprietary)	Prevention and treatment of deficiency and anaemia Prevention of neural tube defects in pregnancy Used in cancer chemotherapy regimens	Involved in cell division, DNA synthesis, and the synthesis of amino acids	[b]
B$_{12}$	Cobalamins (non-proprietary)	Prevention and treatment of deficiency and anaemia	Co-enzyme used in metabolic processes, including DNA synthesis	[b]Deficiency often results from malabsorption and requires parenteral treatment
C	Ascorbic acid (non-proprietary)	Prevention and treatment of deficiency and scurvy	Co-enzyme used in metabolic processes	[b]Deficiency leads to scurvy, which may still be seen in developed countries

MHRA, Medicines and Healthcare Products Regulatory Agency.
[a] Fat-soluble vitamin.
[b] Water-soluble vitamin.

Are they all the same?

Each named vitamin is different and has a different biological function. Vitamins are sometimes grouped according to whether they are water or fat soluble. Fat-soluble vitamins can become deficient in patients with fat malabsorption, and with excessive dosing they may accumulate in the body, which may result in overdose and adverse effects. Vitamins A, D, and E have analogues (several compounds with similar structures that comprise that vitamin). These fat-soluble vitamins may be prescribed in units rather than milligrams because many compounds make up the groups.

What are the notable adverse effects to look out for?

Hypervitaminosis can occur with excessive administration of vitamins, in particular those which are fat soluble (such as A and D). This can lead to effects such as gastrointestinal disturbance and headache as well as liver changes and electrolyte disturbance.

Vitamin A is associated with congenital malformations of the foetus, and vitamin A supplements should generally be avoided during pregnancy. The retinoid derivatives (such as tretinoin and isotretinoin) are contraindicated in pregnancy and effective contraception is a requirement of their use.

Thiamine (vitamin B_1) has been associated with hypersensitivity reactions, particularly when given parenterally (e.g. as Pabrinex® preparations). Long-term use of high-dose pyridoxine (vitamin B_6) may lead to neuropathy.

Other considerations

Multivitamin preparations can be purchased over the counter or prescribed. Multivitamins are often prescribed and/or labelled as 'Vitamins BPC' or 'Multivitamins'.

70 Drugs for Eczema, Psoriasis, and Skin Conditions

Commonly used examples

Emollients, e.g. paraffin, soy bean oil, urea.

Topical steroids, e.g. hydrocortisone, betamethasone (*Betnovate-RD®*), clobetasone (*Eumovate®*), beclometasone, clobetasol (*Dermovate®*).

Dithranol

Vitamin D (and analogues), e.g. calcipotriol, calcitriol, tacalcitol.

Are these drugs all the same?

There is a wide range of dermatological conditions and a range of treatments that can be used to manage them. Their actions and uses are different, and although some agents may be used for a variety of different conditions, some are only used for a specific dermatological condition.

What are these drugs used to treat?

Eczema is an inflammatory disorder resulting in inflammation, drying, and scaling of the skin. It is associated with itching and presents a risk of infection. It is commonly managed with emollients and topical steroids.

Psoriasis can have similar appearance and similar symptoms to eczema but is a distinctly different condition. Psoriasis is caused by an overproduction of skin cells, which presents as plaques or pustules on the surface of the skin that can be itchy, painful, and disfiguring. It is typically managed using emollients and vitamin D preparations, although a range of other treatments such as biologic medicines, and phototherapy may also be used.

What do these drugs do?

Emollients

Emollients are used to help the skin retain moisture and reverse the symptoms of the dermatological condition.

Topical steroids

Many skin conditions, including eczema, are either caused by, or involve, inflammatory processes. Steroids are powerful drugs that can be very effective in reducing the underlying inflammation. Topical administration allows them to be used effectively whilst minimising adverse effects. In severe cases systemic doses may be given.

Rapid Medicines Management for Healthcare Professionals, First Edition. Paul Deslandes, Simon Young and Ben Pitcher.
© 2020 John Wiley & Sons Ltd. Published 2020 by John Wiley & Sons Ltd.

Anti-infective agents
The skin itself can be infected by pathogens such as bacteria or fungi. This can be a common secondary problem in patients with eczema or other skin conditions that cause breaks in the skin. Anti-infective agents help to eradicate the pathogen responsible for the infection.

Combinations
Some dermatological preparations are formulated as combination products. Common examples included the combination of anti-infective agents and steroids (e.g. Daktacort®, which combines hydrocortisone and miconazole).

What's the difference between different types?
Emollients
Emollients occlude the skin's surface to prevent loss of moisture. This is generally achieved by applying some form of oil to the skin, commonly a petroleum derivative such as paraffin wax. Some emollients are based on plant products such as soy bean oil (e.g. Balneum®). Emollients are formulated into lotions and creams to balance the oily/greasy active ingredient with a product that is more acceptable to the patient. Emollients may be added to soaps and shampoos but this has been seen to be of limited benefit. Some emollients contain added ingredients such as urea (intended to soften the keratin in scaly skin), coal tar (intended to reduce the proliferation of keratinocytes in psoriasis) or plant extracts such as oatmeal (Aveeno®).

Topical steroids
Topical steroids have the same pharmacodynamics as steroids administered by any other route (see Chapter 65), inhibiting various inflammatory processes and stimulating other anti-inflammatory pathways.

Treatments for psoriasis
Treatments such as dithranol disrupt the ability of mitochondria to provide energy to the cell; this slows the excessive production of skin cells, which causes the psoriatic plaques.

Vitamin D analogues are believed to modulate the ability of the cells to proliferate and therefore prevent the development of plaques.

Anti-infective agents
The mechanisms of antibiotics and antifungal drugs used in dermatology are as the same as those used in other therapeutic arenas. These are further discussed in Chapters 60 and 61.

How are these drugs given?
Many drugs given for the treatment of skin conditions can be applied topically to the affected area on the surface of the skin. Some drugs (such as steroids) may also be administered systemically, although this may result in systemic adverse effects. The respective benefits and drawbacks of topical administration are discussed in Chapter 18.

Dosing
Fingertip units
Fingertip units (FTUs) provide guidance on how much cream should be applied to an area of the body to ensure appropriate dosing whatever the size of the patient. An FTU is the

quantity of cream that is squeezed onto an adult's fingertip from the crease of the first knuckle to the tip of the finger (this is discussed in more depth in Chapter 18).

Emollients

Emollients need to be applied regularly and in large quantities. The amount applied varies from product to product. There is no pharmacologically active ingredient in emollients and overdosing is not a concern; there is greater risk in undertreating than overtreating. It is commonly recommended to apply emollients at least three to four times a day.

Topical steroids

In contrast to the emollients, topical steroids should be applied sparingly. This is especially true of the stronger formulations, which are capable of causing systemic side effects such as adrenal suppression. Clinically, the lowest strength of steroid which is still fully effective should be used. The most potent steroid creams should only be used when directed by a specialist.

The *British National Formulary* categorises topical steroids by potency. The mildest topical steroids can be bought over the counter without prescription, whilst the most potent are only recommended for short-term use under supervision of a specialist.

Mild, e.g. hydrocortisone.
Moderate, e.g. Betnovate-RD®, Clobetasone (Eumovate®).
Potent, e.g. beclometasone.
Very potent, e.g. Dermovate®.

Tubes of topical steroid will note the type of drug and the concentration of drug in the form of a percentage. Whilst a higher percentage of drug does mean a stronger preparation, it is important to remember that the difference in strength between mild and moderately mild steroids is far greater than a small increase in percentage (i.e. 1% hydrocortisone is still considered milder than 0.05% clobetasone).

Different strengths of topical steroid are required depending on the severity of the condition being treated and the location on the body. Stronger steroids are required to treat areas of the body which have thicker skin, such as the soles of the feet. Areas of the body with thinner skin, such as the face or groin, require weaker steroids.

What are the notable adverse effects to look out for?
Emollients

- Emollients can leave the skin covered in oily residue. This can feel greasy for the patient and can stain clothing and bedsheets.
- The oily covering provided by emollients can block hair follicles and cause folliculitis.

Topical steroids

As the cream is applied locally most of the side effects are seen at or around the site of application. This can include thinning of the skin, irritation, and increased hair growth. As steroids are an immunosuppressant, if the affected skin is infected the topical steroid may actually slow healing and allow the infection to spread.

Treatments for psoriasis

Dithranol tends to stain the skin (and clothing) brown.

How can the adverse effects be minimised?
Emollients
Emollients are generally formulated as creams or ointments. Whilst these two types contain the same key ingredients, ointments contain a greater proportion of oil, which makes them more effective in occluding the surface of the skin but also makes them less palatable to patients.

Creams are less oily and feel like they are absorbed more easily, leaving the skin dry and avoiding some of the unpleasant after effects.

The risk of folliculitis can be reduced by applying to the skin in the direction of hair growth (i.e. from the top of the arm down towards the hand or from the knee down towards the foot).

Topical steroids
To avoid adverse effects the lowest strength of steroid which is still fully effective should be used. The most potent steroid creams should only be used when directed by a specialist.

It is important to remember that the adverse effect profile of topical steroids is actually quite mild. Patients may need to be reassured of this as the impact of the adverse effects of these agents is far less than the impact of undertreating the eczema, yet fear of adverse effects is a leading cause of non-compliance.

Other considerations
Keeping it clean
The large quantities of emollient which are dispensed and administered are typically supplied in a tub or a 'pump dispenser'. Whilst the tub makes it easier to access the emollient it presents a potential hazard. When the patient (or healthcare professional) puts their hand into the tub they introduce bacteria into the emollient. Bacteria can grow and multiply in the medication and it is therefore possible to inadvertently spread bacteria over the patient and infect broken skin. To help prevent this emollient should be removed from the tub using a clean spoon or spatula before being applied to the patient.

71 Non-steroidal Anti-inflammatory Drugs

Commonly used examples
Non selective. Aspirin, diclofenac, ibuprofen, indomethacin, naproxen, piroxicam.
COX-1 selective. Flurbiprofen, ketorolac.
COX-2 selective. Celecoxib, etoricoxib, meloxicam.

Are these drugs all the same?
Non-steroidal anti-inflammatory drugs (NSAIDs) can be divided into broad groups according to their mechanism of action. Drugs from the same group typically have similar pharmacodynamic properties and adverse effects, but drugs from different groups may vary.

What are these drugs used to treat?
NSAIDs are most commonly used to treat pain and inflammation associated with musculoskeletal disorders and other conditions (including peri-operatively). They are also given to treat pyrexia. Low doses of aspirin are used to inhibit platelet aggregation in people with a high risk of stroke or myocardial infarction (see Chapter 40).

What do these drugs do?
NSAIDs inhibit the cyclooxygenase enzymes that mediate the production of prostanoids. Prostanoids are a group of inflammatory mediators that includes prostaglandins, prostacyclin, and thromboxane. Prostanoids exert a number of physiological effects in the body, including vasodilatation and enhanced vascular permeability (resulting in swelling), sensitisation of nociceptive receptors (leading to an increased response to painful stimuli), and alteration in thermoregulatory mechanisms in the hypothalamus (leading to fever). By inhibiting the production of these compounds, NSAIDs have anti-inflammatory, analgesic, and antipyretic properties.

In addition to these roles, prostaglandins also mediate other effects within the body. These include promoting the secretion of gastro protective mucus, facilitating and inhibiting platelet aggregation, and facilitating blood flow and natriuresis in the kidney. Disruption of these effects by NSAIDs can lead to adverse drug reactions.

What's the difference between different types?
NSAIDs from the different groups exert their effects in slightly different ways. All NSAIDs inhibit cyclooxygenase (COX) enzymes in the body. However, cyclooxygenase is present in two different forms (COX-1 and COX-2). Whilst some NSAIDs inhibit both forms to a similar

Rapid Medicines Management for Healthcare Professionals, First Edition. Paul Deslandes, Simon Young and Ben Pitcher.
© 2020 John Wiley & Sons Ltd. Published 2020 by John Wiley & Sons Ltd.

extent, certain NSAIDs preferentially inhibit one form of the enzyme over the other, which can create a different side effect profile. Whilst there is some limited evidence to indicate that certain NSAIDs might be more effective than others, there is clearer evidence that adverse effects vary, reflecting these subtle pharmacodynamic differences.

How are these drugs given?

NSAIDs are available in a number of different formulations, allowing administration via a number of different routes and for different indications:

By mouth, regularly (up to four times day) or as required, to treat chronic inflammatory illnesses, acute pain, and pyrexia.
Rectally, regularly (usually daily) or as required, to treat chronic inflammatory illnesses, acute pain, and pyrexia.
Topically regularly (usually three to four times a day) or as required, to treat chronic inflammatory illnesses or acute localised pain.
By eye, regularly (usually two to four times a day), for prophylaxis and reduction of inflammation following ocular surgery. By eye, regularly, prior to ocular surgery to prevent miosis.
Parenterally for the short-term treatment of acute and post-operative pain.

Dosing

NSAIDs should generally be prescribed at the lowest possible dose, for the shortest possible duration necessary to control pain, inflammation, or pyrexia. This is intended to reduce the risk of serious adverse drug reactions.

What are the notable adverse effects to look out for?

Common side effects include nausea, vomiting, dyspepsia, diarrhoea, headache, dizziness, and rash.
NSAIDs may also be more rarely associated with severe adverse effects which may be fatal.

Gastrointestinal

The gastro protective prostaglandins are primarily synthesised through the action of COX-1, therefore NSAIDs, which inhibit this form of the enzyme, can cause gastrointestinal adverse effects such as dyspepsia and peptic ulceration. Whilst COX-2 selective inhibitors are less likely to cause these adverse effects, COX-2 plays a role in ulcer healing, and COX-2 selective NSAIDs are contra-indicated in patients with active gastrointestinal bleeding. Hypersensitivity reactions (including anaphylaxis and rashes) as well as bronchospasm and worsening of asthma may also occur.

Cardiovascular

Thrombotic events such as myocardial infarction and stroke are known adverse effects, particularly of COX-2 inhibitors. Although less common than gastrointestinal symptoms, these effects have led to the withdrawal from the market of certain COX-2 selective inhibitors (e.g. rofecoxib). However, cardiovascular events appear to be a dose-related adverse effect of many commonly used NSAIDs (including ibuprofen) and caution is required.

Renal

NSAIDs can reduce the excretion of sodium and water from the kidney, resulting in fluid retention, increased blood pressure, and worsening of heart failure. Altered renal perfusion may lead to acute kidney injury.

How can the adverse effects be minimised?

NSAIDs should generally be prescribed at the lowest possible dose, for the shortest possible duration in order to minimise adverse effects.

Medicines such as histamine H_2 receptor antagonists and proton pump inhibitors, which reduce gastric acid secretion, have been shown to reduce the incidence of NSAID-induced peptic ulceration. Misoprostol (a synthetic prostaglandin analogue) is available as combination tablets with certain NSAIDs (e.g. arthrotec) and also protects against peptic ulceration. However, it is less well tolerated than proton pump inhibitors. Non-selective NSAIDs are contraindicated in patients with a history of gastrointestinal bleeding and COX-2 selective NSAIDs should be used with caution.

Non-selective NSAIDs should be used with caution and COX-2 selective inhibitors avoided in patients with a history of ischaemic heart disease, cerebrovascular disease, and peripheral arterial disease due to the risk of thrombotic events.

All NSAIDs should be used with caution or avoided in patients with renal impairment.

What drug interactions are important?

There is an increased risk of bleeding when NSAIDs (particularly non-selective and COX-1 inhibitors) are given with anticoagulants, antiplatelet medicines (including clopidogrel and aspirin), or selective serotonin re-uptake inhibitor and serotonin and noradrenaline reuptake inhibitor antidepressants.

NSAIDs reduce the renal excretion of certain medicines such as lithium and methotrexate, which can lead to severe toxicity.

As a result of causing sodium and water retention, NSAIDs can counteract the effects of antihypertensive medication and worsen heart failure. NSAIDs can reduce the effectiveness of diuretics. NSAID use in combination with angiotensin converting enzyme inhibitors, angiotensin receptor blockers or diuretics may increase the risk of renal failure.

It is important to consider the possibility that a patient is taking over-the-counter NSAIDs when assessing the potential for drug interactions.

Other considerations

Although commonly prescribed in both primary and secondary care and available over the counter from pharmacies, NSAIDs are a common contributory factor in hospital admissions and care in their usage is required.

Clinical note: other drugs affecting eicosanoid pharmacology

Whilst NSAIDs inhibit the synthesis of prostaglandins, thereby reducing their inflammatory effects, a number of other drugs are prostaglandin analogues or act as prostaglandin receptor agonists and are used in a range of different conditions. These include misoprostol (mentioned above), which can attenuate some of the gastrointestinal adverse effects of NSAIDs and which is also used in termination of pregnancy. Other prostaglandin receptor agonists include bimatoprost, latanoprost, and tafluprost, which are formulated as eyedrops and used in the management of glaucoma. Iloprost is formulated as a nebuliser solution and used for the treatment of pulmonary hypertension.

Other drugs inhibiting the effects of eicosanoids are the leukotriene receptor antagonists montelukast and zafirlukast. These oral preparations help to reduce the inflammation associated with asthma and are used as add-on therapy to inhaled corticosteroids.

72 Local Anaesthetics

These drugs provide pain relief or numbing of an area.

Commonly used examples

Lidocaine (lignocaine).
Prilocaine.
Bupivacaine.

Are these drugs all the same?

Local anaesthetics have similar mechanisms of action, but they can have different durations of action, can be administered by different routes, and can sometimes be combined with other agents, such as adrenaline.

What are these drugs used to treat?

Local anaesthetics can be used to numb an area prior to a potentially painful procedure such as suturing a wound or a dental procedure, or to reduce the pain of injured or inflamed tissue. They can also be used in a spinal block, numbing all sensation below its point of insertion in the spine. The most well-known example of this is its use in childbirth, but this can also be used to facilitate surgical procedures without the need for general anaesthetic.

Lidocaine may be administered systemically to treat cardiac arrhythmias.

What do these drugs do?

Painful stimuli are detected by specific receptors (termed nociceptors) found in the skin and other tissues. Stimulation of these receptors results in the conduction of nerve impulses (signals) to the brain, where they are recognised and experienced as pain. Local anaesthetics reduce pain by interrupting the transmission of these nerve signals (largely through an effect on the movement of sodium ions across the cell membrane). If the signals do not reach the brain, then pain will not be experienced. Local anaesthetics have no impact on the injury or inflammation itself, only on the patient's ability to feel it.

What's the difference between different types?

Local anaesthetics tend to share the same mechanism of action. However, some (e.g. bupivacaine) have a slower onset and longer duration of action, whilst others (e.g. lidocaine) have a quicker onset and shorter duration of action. There are also differences in their potential to cause cardiac toxicity.

Rapid Medicines Management for Healthcare Professionals, First Edition. Paul Deslandes, Simon Young and Ben Pitcher.
© 2020 John Wiley & Sons Ltd. Published 2020 by John Wiley & Sons Ltd.

Some local anaesthetics are combined with vasoconstrictors (such as adrenaline/epinephrine). The vasoconstrictor reduces the flow of blood through the tissue, increasing the duration of action and reducing the risk of toxicity. This can also help reduce bleeding if the agent is being used to numb a wound or incision site.

How are these drugs given?

Local anaesthetics can be administered by a variety of routes but are typically applied directly to the intended site of action (locally) via routes such as subcutaneous injection, topical creams or patches, or sprays. They can also be injected directly into the spine as part of an epidural.

Whilst there are certain circumstances where it is done, it is unusual and potentially dangerous to administer local anaesthetics systemically by the intravenous route. Small amounts of local anaesthetic may be administered orally to act locally on a painful throat.

Dosing

The dosing of local anaesthetics can be somewhat variable depending on the size of the area that needs to be anaesthetised, the route of administration, and the patient's weight. The greater the amount administered, the greater the risk of toxicity, a problem enhanced in smaller patients and mitigated by administering the local anaesthetic with a vasoconstrictor.

What are the notable adverse effects to look out for?

In normal usage the most common adverse effect is a total loss of sensation (not only pain but touch and temperature) at the site of administration. This is because the local anaesthetic will interfere with the function of many types of nerves not only those that conduct painful stimuli.

If the local anaesthetic disperses away from the site of administration, it can start to affect other organs and systems. Its ability to interfere with normal function of nerves can have a potentially dangerous impact on the central nervous system and the heart.

Low levels of toxicity will cause dizziness, drowsiness, and arrhythmias. If toxicity continues to increase the patient can experience cardiac arrest, respiratory failure, and loss of consciousness. If a patient who has been administered a local anaesthetic begins demonstrating symptoms of toxicity, it should be immediately discontinued and the patient fully assessed.

How can the adverse effects be minimised?

Risk of toxicity can be reduced through careful administration. This is particularly important when administering via subcutaneous injection where it is important (as with all subcutaneous injections) to ensure that the needle does not enter a vein, resulting in accidental intravenous administration.

Risk of toxicity can also be reduced by combining the local anaesthetic with a vasoconstrictor such as adrenaline (this is usually provided as a premixed solution). When combined with a vasoconstrictor, significantly higher doses can be given with a reduced risk of toxicity.

What needs to be monitored?

Whilst these drugs are generally well tolerated, it is always prudent to keep in mind the potential for systemic adverse effects and report them immediately.

What drug interactions are important?

The potential for cardiovascular adverse effects can be increased by combining local anaesthetics with other drugs that act on the heart, such as beta-blockers, calcium channel blockers, and angiotensin converting enzyme inhibitors.

73 Blank Therapeutics Chapter Template

Dear reader, if there is a drug or group of drugs that we had not included in the book, but which are relevant to your practice, please use this blank template to compile pertinent information for your professional development and learning. Please see Chapter 32 for an explanation of how we have used the headings.

Commonly used examples

Are these drugs all the same?

What are these drugs used to treat?

What do these drugs do?

What's the difference between different types?

How are these drugs given?

Rapid Medicines Management for Healthcare Professionals, First Edition. Paul Deslandes, Simon Young and Ben Pitcher.
© 2020 John Wiley & Sons Ltd. Published 2020 by John Wiley & Sons Ltd.

Dosing

What are the notable adverse effects to look out for?

How can the adverse effects be minimised?

What needs to be monitored?

What drug interactions are important?

Discontinuing treatment

Other considerations

Practice Considerations

74 Vaccinations

Vaccination

Vaccination is the most effective method of preventing infectious disease and has allowed infectious diseases such as smallpox to be eradicated worldwide. Many other diseases which caused severe morbidity and mortality, such as polio and tetanus, have also been eliminated from much of the globe because of vaccination programmes. The majority of vaccines are administered to prevent disease but it is a method that can be used to attenuate a disease after it has been contracted.

Vaccination is the name given to the *physical act* of administering material which possesses antigenic properties to stimulate the immune system to develop immunity to a pathogen. The resulting physiological process of *inducing an immune response* as a method of 'pump priming' the immune system is termed immunisation.

Immunisation

The process of inducing an immune response as a method of 'pump priming' the immune system with an immunogenic material to protect against infectious disease is termed immunisation.

Vaccine types

Vaccine science is incredibly complex but there are four basic 'vaccine types':

1. Live attenuated vaccines
   Live vaccines use a weakened (attenuated) form of the germ that causes a disease. The immunogenic material is very similar to the natural infection; this means the immune response is long lasting and strongly provoked. One or two doses often give lifetime protection against the infectious disease.
   Examples
   MMR, smallpox, and chickenpox.
2. Inactivated vaccines
   These are 'killed' versions of the infectious agent. The protection they provide is not as robust as live vaccines so booster doses are needed over a given time schedule in order to sustain immunity.
   Examples
   Hepatitis A, polio, and rabies.
3. Subunit, recombinant, polysaccharide, and conjugate vaccines
   These vaccine types use specific 'chunks' of the infectious agent to provoke the response, such as proteins and sugars that specifically define that germ. As with the inactivated vaccines, their protection is not as robust as live vaccines so 'booster' doses are needed over a given time schedule in order to sustain immunity.

Rapid Medicines Management for Healthcare Professionals, First Edition. Paul Deslandes, Simon Young and Ben Pitcher.
© 2020 John Wiley & Sons Ltd. Published 2020 by John Wiley & Sons Ltd.

Examples
Hib, hepatitis B, and HPV.
4. Toxoid vaccines
   These vaccines use a toxin from the infectious agent that causes the disease to provoke the immunogenic response. The immune response is then raised against the toxoid and prevents its effects (the target is not the microbe itself).
   Examples
   Diphtheria and tetanus.

Each vaccine type has its own set of indications and contraindications, e.g. live vaccines may not be suitable for some immunocompromised patients. There is specific information available to healthcare professionals for vaccination of specialist groups, e.g. healthcare workers, pregnant women, and people with long-term health conditions. Immunisation schedules can vary or particular schedules may be required in certain medical conditions, such as post-splenectomy. Another area of impact upon healthcare professionals is that of travel vaccinations. The data that inform the requirements for travel vaccination are constantly changing and consulting the most up-to-date advice is important. This can be obtained from a variety of sources, including pharmacies and specialist travel clinics.

UK 2018 immunisation schedule (this schedule is subject to constant updating)
At age 2 months
DTaP/IPV(polio)/Hib/HepB (diphtheria, tetanus, pertussis (whooping cough), polio, *Haemophilus influenzae* type b and hepatitis B) six-in-one injection (Infanrix hexa®), plus
   PCV (pneumococcal conjugate vaccine) in a separate injection (Prevenar 13®).
   Rotavirus (Rotarix®), oral route (drops).
   Meningitis B (Bexsero®).

At age 3 months
DTaP/IPV(polio)/Hib/HepB six-in-one injection, second dose (Infanrix hexa®), plus
   Rotavirus (Rotarix®), oral route (drops).

At age 4 months
DTaP/IPV(polio)/Hib/HepB six-in-one injection, third dose (Infanrix hexa®), plus
   PCV second dose (Prevenar 13®) in a separate injection.
   Meningitis B, second dose (Bexsero®).

Between 12 and 13 months
Hib/MenC (combined as one injection), fourth dose of Hib and first dose of MenC (Menitorix®), plus
   MMR (measles, mumps, and rubella) combined as one injection (Priorix® or M-M-RVAXPRO®), plus
   PCV third dose (Prevenar 13®) in a separate injection.
   Meningitis B, third dose (Bexsero®).

At age 2 to 8 years
Nasal flu spray annually (Fluenz®). For children aged 2, 3, and 4, this is usually given in the GP surgery. Children in school years 1, 2, and 3 may have this at school.

At age 3 years and 4 months
Preschool booster of DTaP/IPV(polio) four-in-one injection (Repevax® or Infanrix-IPV®), plus
   MMR, second dose (Priorix® or M-M-RVAXPRO®) in a separate injection.

At age 12 to 13 years (girls)

HPV (human papillomavirus types 16 and 18), two injections (Gardasil®). The second injection is given 6–12 months after the first one.

At age 14 years

Td/IPV(polio) booster three-in-one injection (Revaxis®).

Men ACWY: combined protection against meningitis A, C, W, and Y (Nimenrix® or Menveo®).

Adult

Influenza (annual) and PPV (pneumococcal polysaccharide vaccine): for those aged over 65 years and those in high-risk groups.

Td/IPV(polio): for those not fully immunised as a child (Revaxis®).

DTaP/IPV: for pregnant women from 20 weeks of gestation to protect the newborn baby against whooping cough (Boostrix-IPV® or Repevax®).

Shingles (Zostavax®) vaccine: for adults aged 70 years (plus catch-up for adults aged 78 and 79).

This vaccination schedule is simplified from *Immunisation against infectious disease*, which outlines in detail the principles, practice, and procedures of immunisation and the diseases against which vaccination schedules are used in clinical practice in the UK.

https://www.gov.uk/government/collections/immunisation-against-infectious-disease-the-green-book#the-green-book

Herd immunity

Herd immunity arises when a high proportion of a population is protected against a virus or bacteria by a vaccination programme. This makes it difficult for a disease to spread because there are very few susceptible people left to infect. Herd immunity can help to protect those who have not been vaccinated due to either being too young or because of ill-health. If the number of people receiving vaccinations drops then herd immunity may be lost and vulnerable individuals may be at risk of infection.

Anti-vax

In recent years, misplaced concerns over the safety of vaccines have resulted in a drop in childhood vaccination rates. This has placed children at greater risk of infection and reduced herd immunity. Whilst vaccines do have the potential for causing undesirable effects (as any medication can), the risk is greatly outweighed by the benefit, and assertions that they can cause long-term developmental disorders (such as autism spectrum disorder) are not supported by evidence.

75 Antimicrobial Stewardship

What is an antimicrobial drug?

An antimicrobial drug is one that is used to treat an infection caused by a pathogenic micro-organism such as a bacterium, fungus, or virus.

What is antimicrobial resistance?

Antimicrobial resistance describes a situation where a micro-organism is no longer sensitive to (i.e. it has been killed or its growth inhibited by) an antimicrobial drug. Infections caused by resistant micro-organisms will therefore be more difficult to treat, with the potential for increased morbidity and mortality. One of the best-known examples of antimicrobial resistance is the *Staphylococcus aureus* bacterium with resistance to the antibacterial drug methicillin (methicillin-resistant *Staphylococcus aureus* or MRSA). However, resistance of other types of micro-organism to a number of different antimicrobial drugs is a significant concern.

What are the consequences of antimicrobial resistance?

If micro-organisms can no longer be killed by antimicrobial drugs, this can have potentially severe implications for both patients and the healthcare system more widely. An estimate from 2016 suggested that approximately 700 000 deaths globally could be attributed to antimicrobial-resistant infections.

If patients experience infections caused by organisms that are resistant to commonly used antimicrobial drugs, they may need to be given second-line drugs. These may be associated with more severe adverse effects for the patient and greater cost for the healthcare service. In the worst-case scenario, if an infection cannot be treated with any drug, the patient may not survive. Treatment of resistant infections may require hospital admission or result in prolonged inpatient treatment, with associated cost implications.

The potential for resistant infections may also increase the risk associated with some common medical interventions, making them no longer safe. Treatments that impair the immune response, such as cancer chemotherapy, immunosuppressant drugs used in conditions such as rheumatoid arthritis, and following organ transplantation, as well as surgical procedures, could no longer be used.

What is the mechanism underlying antimicrobial resistance?

A proportion of micro-organisms will have a natural defence mechanism that protects them against the effects of a given antimicrobial drug, and as a result they will not be killed by it. A common example is bacteria that are resistant to penicillins. Some bacteria are able to

Rapid Medicines Management for Healthcare Professionals, First Edition. Paul Deslandes, Simon Young and Ben Pitcher.
© 2020 John Wiley & Sons Ltd. Published 2020 by John Wiley & Sons Ltd.

produce an enzyme (known as beta-lactamase) that alters the penicillin molecule, making it inactive. Furthermore, following exposure to an antimicrobial, some micro-organisms will be able to change and adapt to prevent the drug from working. When these organisms replicate, the ability to resist the effects of the antimicrobial will be passed on to the next generation. Whilst susceptible organisms are killed, the resistant ones will remain and form the basis of a resistant infection.

What contributes to antimicrobial resistance?

One of the main drivers of antimicrobial resistance is the overuse of antimicrobial agents. The more micro-organisms are exposed to antimicrobial drugs, the more likely it is that resistant organisms will survive and pass on their resistance via 'survival of the fittest'. The widespread use of antimicrobials for minor self-limiting infections and their indiscriminate use in agriculture have driven the increased development of antimicrobial resistance.

How can antimicrobial resistance be reduced?

One of the effective approaches to minimise antimicrobial resistance is the more judicious use of antimicrobial drugs. The strategy to achieve this is commonly known as 'antimicrobial stewardship'. Antimicrobial stewardship takes a system-wide approach to the use of antimicrobial drugs, with the aim of maintaining their future effectiveness. Details of National Institute for Health and Care Excellence guidance on antimicrobial stewardship can be found in their guideline NG15. Key principles include the monitoring of resistance patterns and antimicrobial prescribing, education for healthcare professionals, and audit of processes. When antimicrobials are prescribed, the shortest effective course should be used and, depending on the treatment context, microbiological samples taken to guide treatment choice. This may include a move away from the traditional idea that patients should be told to 'complete the course', and instead discontinue treatment once symptoms have resolved.

Another important mechanism to reduce the spread of resistant organisms is the use of effective infection control procedures. Standard precautions to be applied to the care of all patients (whether or not there is evidence of infection) can help to reduce the transfer of microorganisms from one person to another. Standard precautions include the use of hand hygiene between contact with each patient and protective equipment such as gloves, gowns, and masks. The appropriate cleaning and sterilisation of reusable equipment and the safe disposal of single-use equipment (particularly needles and other medical sharps) is essential.

Antimicrobial drug development

The development of new antimicrobials for resistant infections is challenging and has resulted in a limited number of new drugs coming to the market. The number of patients with an infection caused by a given resistant strain may be limited, making it difficult to recruit an adequate number of participants to clinical trials. There is also significant financial risk to pharmaceutical companies. As the drug goes through the development process, it is possible that resistant organisms will emerge, making the drug obsolete before it even reaches the market. If the drug does reach the market, it is likely to be reserved for limited use in particular situations. It is therefore unlikely to represent a viable financial prospect with return on the significant investment needed to bring it to market. Alternative strategies to the usual drug development model may be required to overcome these hurdles.

76 Substance Misuse

Healthcare professionals with responsibility for managing medicines should be aware of the impact of the misuse of substances on the efficacy and safety of medication and consequently upon the well-being of the patient under their care.

A range of substances can be misused and the contexts in which those substances are misused vary widely. A range of circumstances and the considerations for the healthcare professional are outlined below. This list is illustrative and the precise nature of possible substance misuse in patients under your care should be considered.

The misuse of non-medicinal substances

There are many ways of classifying misused substances. There are overlaps between the categories below. Some of these substances are legal and others are illegal, and this is dependent on the country in which they are consumed, and in some cases the age of the user.

Central nervous system (CNS) stimulants. Legal substances in this category in the UK include caffeine and nicotine. Illegal substances in this category (unless they are prescribed for a medicinal purpose) include amphetamines and cocaine. Stimulants are broadly misused for the high that they produce. As well as the 'rush' that stimulants produce they are also used to produce a 'wakefulness' effect. The widespread use of caffeine illustrates the importance of considering the use of substances that are legal. Substances such as dexamfetamine may be misused to aid focus and attention (a crossover with a therapeutic effect).

Hallucinogens are a group of substances that distort reality. There are very few medicinal uses of the hallucinogens at present. Examples of hallucinogens include lysergic acid diethylamide (LSD), psilocybin (obtained from mushrooms), and mescaline. These substances may make a user feel, hear, or see things that don't exist. They are used for the pleasure derived from their effects and also to promote and stimulate creativity.

Depressants slow down or inhibit the CNS (brain, spinal cord, nerves). CNS depressants are prescribed to help people with conditions such as anxiety (either as a generalised disorder or associated with depression and other conditions). These drugs make the consumer feel sleepy and light-headed. Examples include alcohol, barbiturates, and benzodiazepines.

Narcotics are substances that are used to relieve pain and or induce sleepiness. They can be misused to induce euphoria (e.g. the opioids) or for their soporific effect (e.g. cannabis).

Other substances are also misused for combinations of these effects, examples include inhalants (e.g. acetone, aerosol propellants found in spray paints, cleaning fluids, and freons). Amyl nitrite is misused for its psychoactive effect and is a popular recreational drug in the gay community. Of more recent concern are substances such as Spice (a synthetic cannabinoid) and other so-called 'legal highs' which were made illegal by the Psychoactive Substances Act 2016. The legal highs are more properly termed novel/new psychoactive substances.

Rapid Medicines Management for Healthcare Professionals, First Edition. Paul Deslandes, Simon Young and Ben Pitcher.
© 2020 John Wiley & Sons Ltd. Published 2020 by John Wiley & Sons Ltd.

The misuse of licensed medication (prescription and non-prescription medication)

A range of prescription and non-prescription drugs have the potential to be misused and includes general sale list medicines, pharmacy-only medicines, prescription-only medicines, and controlled drug (CD) categories. All of the drugs that are CDs are classified as such because of potentially harmful outcomes resulting from misuse. Medications such as cyclizine (an antihistamine used for nausea and vomiting), procyclidine (used to manage the side effects of antipsychotics), gabapentin, pregabalin, tramadol, and insulin are known to be misused.

Some of the most commonly misused over-the-counter (OTC) drugs are:

1. *Codeine-based medicines, e.g. co-codamol.* These are repeatedly purchased and consumed by misusers for the small amount of codeine that is present in the product. The codeine in co-codamol products is metabolised to morphine and its addictive properties result in physical dependence.
2. *Dextromethorphan.* Dextromethorphan is found in some OTC cough preparations. It has sedative, dissociative, and stimulant properties (at lower doses). It may be combined (by misusers) with sedating antihistamines for their soporific effect.
3. *Sedative antihistamines.* Patients often start taking these medicines to treat insomnia and find they cannot stop. Regular use leads to tolerance and the dose taken needs to be increased to maintain the effect.
4. *Decongestants.* Decongestants such as pseudoephedrine are sympathetic nervous system stimulants and are pharmacologically related to the amphetamines. They may be taken for the 'buzz' that users feel on consumption. They have also been purchased OTC and used as precursors to the manufacture of the stimulant methamphetamine (crystal meth).
5. Laxatives tend to be misused as a pharmacological tool for weight loss. They are often misused by those with eating disorders.

Important definitions
Tolerance
Tolerance is defined as a person's diminished response to a drug as a result of repeated use. People can develop tolerance to both illicit drugs and prescription medications. Tolerance is a physical effect of repeated use of a drug, not necessarily a sign of addiction. For example, patients with chronic pain may develop tolerance to some effects of prescription pain medications without developing an addiction to them.

Dependence
The words *dependence* and *addiction* are often used interchangeably, but there are important differences between the two. In medical terms, dependence specifically refers to a physical condition in which *the body has adapted to the presence of a drug*. If an individual with drug dependence stops taking that drug suddenly, that person will experience predictable and measurable symptoms, known as withdrawal syndrome.

Addiction
According to the National Institute on Drug Abuse, addiction is a 'chronic, relapsing brain disease that is characterized by compulsive drug seeking and use, despite harmful consequences'. In other words, addiction is an uncontrollable or overwhelming need to use a drug, and this compulsion is long-lasting and can return unexpectedly after a period of improvement.

77 Medicines Licensing and Classification

Before a medicine can be made available for routine prescribing, it must be granted marketing authorisation by the appropriate licensing body. In the UK, the Medicines and Healthcare Products Regulatory Agency (MHRA) is the licensing authority, whilst there are equivalent organisations in Europe (the European Medicines Agency) and in the United States of America (US Food and Drug Administration, FDA). In order to receive marketing authorisation, the medicine must be shown to safe, effective, and of good quality, a concept formally introduced in the UK Medicines Act 1968.

Marketing authorisation

If the criteria of safety, efficacy, and good quality are met, a medicine can be granted marketing authorisation. The marketing authorisation specifies how the medicine can be used in practice, for example outlining the indications, dosage etc. This information is contained in the Summary of Product Characteristics (SmPC) for the medicine. For most medicines, the SmPC can be found via the website www.medicines.org.uk.

'Off label' use of a medicine

In some instances, medicines may be used outside the conditions specified in their marketing authorisation. Such usage is typically termed 'off label' and may include use of the medicine for a different indication or at a different dose to that specified in the SmPC. Use in this way is common in certain medical specialties such as paediatrics, where it is difficult to conduct clinical trials. Whilst it is not unlawful to prescribe a medicine outside its marketing authorisation, it does place additional responsibility on the healthcare professionals involved. Advice for healthcare professionals in this area is available through regulatory bodies such as the General Medical Council.

Unlicensed medicines

For the treatment of certain conditions, or for certain patients, a licensed medicine may not be available or may have been tried but proven to be ineffective. In these circumstances it may be possible to use an unlicensed medicine instead. Unlicensed medicines will not have been reviewed by the licensing authority, therefore it is more difficult to assess their safety, efficacy, and quality. As with off-label usage, healthcare professionals have additional responsibilities when using these medicines. Before prescribing an unlicensed medicine, the prescriber should ensure that there is no suitable licensed alternative and that sufficient evidence supports the use of the unlicensed medicine.

Rapid Medicines Management for Healthcare Professionals, First Edition. Paul Deslandes, Simon Young and Ben Pitcher.
© 2020 John Wiley & Sons Ltd. Published 2020 by John Wiley & Sons Ltd.

Medicines classification

The Medicines Act 1968, and subsequently the Human Medicines Regulations 2012, identify three classes of medicine in the UK. These are prescription-only medicine (POM), pharmacy-only medicine (P), and general sale list medicine (GSL), and each has differing levels of control relating to their supply. P and GSL medicines can both be bought by the public, either under the supervision of a pharmacist (P) or from appropriate outlets (GSL). They are sometimes referred to as over-the-counter (OTC) medicines. POMs must be supplied in accordance with a prescription issued by an appropriate healthcare practitioner. The categorisation of a medicine is not fixed, and its status may switch from POM to P or P to GSL. This typically occurs for established medicines where there is perceived to be limited risk when supplied without the need for a prescription. Where safety concerns are identified, it is also possible that a medicine may revert to POM status from P or to P from GSL.

Controlled drugs

In addition to the three categories above, certain medicines are also subject to further restrictions under the Misuse of Drugs Act 1971 and the Misuse of Drugs Regulations 2001. The Misuse of Drugs Act classifies drugs into three categories, A (including heroin and cocaine), B (including amphetamine and cannabis), and C (including benzodiazepines and anabolic steroids), and establishes penalties for their illegal possession and supply.

The Misuse of Drugs Regulations divide drugs into five schedules and specifies how these can be used clinically, including how they must be stored, prescribed, dispensed, and destroyed. Schedule 1 drugs include ecstasy and hallucinogens such as lysergic acid diethylamide (LSD) that have no currently identified medical purpose although they may be used in research. A Home Office license is required to possess these substances. Schedule 2 includes strong opioids (e.g. morphine) and cocaine. These medicines are POMs and additional requirements apply to their storage, record keeping, prescription writing, and destruction. Medicines in Schedule 3 (e.g. buprenorphine, temazepam, and phenobarbital) and Schedule 4 part 1 (benzodiazepines) and part 2 (anabolic steroids) are also POMs, but have fewer restrictions than those in Schedule 2. Schedule 5 medicines may be POM or P, and can include lower strength formulations of medicines from other schedules. Drugs may shift from class to class and/or schedule to schedule according to patterns of misuse.

78 Who Can Prescribe and Who Can Administer Medicines?

What is a prescription?

A prescription is an order that allows an authorised healthcare professional such as a pharmacist to make a legal supply of a medicine to an individual patient.

Who can issue a prescription?

In the UK, the Medicines Act 1968 defined doctors, dentists, and veterinary surgeons as 'appropriate practitioners' who could issue a prescription for a medicine (including a prescription-only medicine [POM]) for an individual patient. The Medicines Act also allowed certified midwives to supply certain medicines (including POMs) as part of their professional practice. Other healthcare professionals could not issue a prescription for an individual patient.

For a number of years, the above restrictions remained in place. However, towards the end of the twentieth century, the UK government (and later the devolved governments representing the individual UK nations) reviewed prescribing rights for healthcare professionals. Initially, this allowed prescribing from a limited formulary by district nurses and health visitors.

In the early 2000s, following the publication of the Crown reports, the extension of prescribing rights to other healthcare professionals was implemented in the UK. Initially, this allowed supplementary prescribing by appropriately trained nurses and pharmacists in collaboration with the patient and medical doctor. Responsibility for diagnosing the patient's condition remained with the doctor, but the patient's treatment could be managed by the supplementary prescriber within an agreed clinical management plan. In the period following introduction of supplementary prescribing, there were limitations on the medicines that could be included in the clinical management plan. Controlled drugs and off-licence medicines could not be prescribed, but this restriction was later lifted. Supplementary prescribing was subsequently extended to include other healthcare professionals such as physiotherapists, podiatrists, and radiographers.

In the mid-2000s, prescribing was extended further with the introduction of independent prescribing for appropriately trained nurses and pharmacists. Here, responsibility for the prescribing process from diagnosis to prescription could be managed by the independent (non-medical) prescriber without the need for a clinical management plan. As with the introduction of supplementary prescribing, there were initially some restrictions on the medicines that could be prescribed (such as controlled drugs). However, independent prescribing has continued to evolve, with the lifting of restrictions on the medicines that can be prescribed by nurses and pharmacists, and the introduction of prescribing by other healthcare professionals such as optometrists, physiotherapists, podiatrists, radiographers, and paramedics.

Rapid Medicines Management for Healthcare Professionals, First Edition. Paul Deslandes, Simon Young and Ben Pitcher.
© 2020 John Wiley & Sons Ltd. Published 2020 by John Wiley & Sons Ltd.

Can medicines be supplied without a prescription?

Not all medicines require a prescription to enable them to be supplied or administered to a patient. Many commonly used treatments can be purchased from pharmacies or from other premises (see also Chapter 77), whilst certain medicines can be administered in an emergency with the intention of saving life. In the UK, there are also mechanisms to facilitate the supply of POMs without the need for a prescription under certain circumstances.

Patient group directions (PGDs) allow certain healthcare professionals to supply or administer a medicine to patients who present to them with a specific condition. PGDs are developed by multidisciplinary groups within a healthcare organisation. Factors to be considered include the setting in which PGD will operate, the condition that will be treated, details of the medicine to be supplied, and the type of healthcare professional who would work under the PGD. Once implemented, a process for reviewing and updating the PGD should be in place.

In certain circumstances, a pharmacist can make an emergency supply of a POM to a patient. The emergency supply can be made either at the request of an independent prescriber (in which case a prescription must be provided with 72 hours of the supply being made) or at the request of a patient. In each case the pharmacist must be satisfied that the supply is justified and certain controlled drugs cannot be supplied through this process.

Who can administer drugs?
Legally

Whilst there is significant restriction on who can prescribe or dispense medication, there is little restriction on who can administer medication. This is of course a necessity, otherwise no member of the public would ever be able to administer medication to a family member. However, no matter who is administering a drug it must be appropriately authorised. A POM can only be administered if it has been prescribed by or is used under the direction of a qualified and registered prescriber (although there are exceptions, most notably relating to the supply and administering of drugs such as adrenaline in an emergency).

Within a work environment

Whilst there may be no legal restriction on who can administer medication, most care environments will have a set policy on who is allowed to administer. Historically, the administration of medication was restricted to qualified healthcare professionals. In recent years, the task of administering medications has been delegated to non-qualified staff (e.g. healthcare support workers) and will be part of the role of the nursing associate.

Professionally

Even if you are legally allowed to administer a drug and it is within the remit of your role in the organisation in which you work, you should only administer a drug if you are confident that you have the knowledge and skills to be able to do it safely and effectively.

79 Medicines Storage

Medications are stored with three primary considerations:

1. *To preserve their integrity*. Medicines are products that can deteriorate biologically and chemically. Much in the way that foods have sell-by and use-by dates so medicines have use-by dates as they degrade in the same way.
   Medicines need to be protected from light, oxygen, and moisture; these three factors can cause the serious deterioration of medication. Medication packaging is not only designed for marketing purposes but often has a practical function in protection of the medication. Another important factor that can influence the spoiling of medication is temperature. Most medicines need to be stored below 25 °C but some medications need to be kept in a fridge, which stay at a temperature between 4 and 8 °C. Refrigerated items should not be frozen. They may also deteriorate (or have their shelf life reduced) if left out of the refrigerator for an extended period of time.
2. *To comply with regulations* such as the Humans Medicines Regulations 2012 and the Misuse of Drugs Act 1971. Medicines are classified into legal categories (Chapter 77) that require them to be stored with consideration of their likelihood to cause harm, or to be misused. Many Schedule 2 and Schedule 3 controlled drugs (CDs) must be stored in a locked cupboard in hospitals and pharmacies, although this no longer applies once the medicine has been dispensed to the patient and taken to their home.
3. *To keep them out of reach* of children and others who could come to harm if they accidentally consumed or used them.

Medication storage in the patient's home

The context of care will dictate how medication should be stored. In a patient's own home medications are stored in order to primarily prevent their deterioration and to keep them away from children and animals. Direction for the safe storage of CDs may fall under the remit of the healthcare professional. For example, patients may be directed by their care team to store 'take home' doses of methadone in wooden locked boxes to prevent children gaining access to a potentially lethal substance. Other consideration should include access to CDs where unscrupulous family members, friends, or neighbours may gain unwarranted access to those medicines.

Medication storage in hospital settings
General principles

Medication should be stored at a level of security commensurate with its proposed use and potential risk. There is a healthcare professional who is deemed responsible for the safe storage and use of medicines in any given clinical area. Patients' own medication may be

Rapid Medicines Management for Healthcare Professionals, First Edition. Paul Deslandes, Simon Young and Ben Pitcher.
© 2020 John Wiley & Sons Ltd. Published 2020 by John Wiley & Sons Ltd.

stored in a locker next to their bed for them to access themselves, with a master key available to the nominated responsible healthcare professional.

Certain medicines may require specific storage areas, e.g. CDs should be stored in appropriately unmarked locked cupboards, products for external use should be stored separately from those that will be taken internally, fridges, cupboards for flammable products, considerations of the storage of cytotoxics, etc. Cupboards will typically have their own unique lock and key. Solid dosage forms are usually stored separately from liquid dosage forms. Medications should be kept under lock and key when not in use.

All CDs for stock and discharge, and patients' own CDs should be stored in areas that comply with current regulations. Many clinical areas will have security that exceeds the legislative requirements. CDs should be stored in a separate locked cupboard from all other medicines. The CD cupboard must have its own dedicated key. The key for the CD cupboard should be kept on the person of the appropriate clinician when not in use. This key should be kept separate from other medicine keys.

Storage should be adequate to allow medication to be protected, appropriately selected from the storage area and medication labels should remain undamaged and intact wherever stored. Fridges and freezers should be checked to ensure they are functioning within the temperature range required to store the medication. Adequate records need to be kept. Protocols should be in place if the temperature falls out of range or in case of equipment failure.

Specific protocols are often written for issues such as transferring control of medication from one clinical area to another, storage and disposal of drugs (with specific regulations covering the disposal of CDs) and the management of patients' own drugs.

Medication storage in care home settings

NICE have generated guidance on managing medicines in care homes. Many of the principles applied in a hospital setting also apply in a care home setting.

https://www.nice.org.uk/guidance/sc1/ifp/chapter/storing-and-disposing-of-medicines-in-care-homes#storing-medicines

The outlined storage processes should be audited along with the processes and protocols put in place to ensure the safe administration and disposal of medication.

80 The 5Rs

Medicines can be one of the greatest tools available to a healthcare practitioner to help improve a patient's health and well-being. However, if an incorrect medicine is given or the correct medicine is given incorrectly there is the potential to cause tremendous harm. Whilst all those involved in the prescribing and administration of medicines should be suitably trained, it is still possible for errors to occur. A strength of having multiple individuals involved in this process (i.e. the practitioner who administers a medicine is not normally the same practitioner who prescribed it) is that the details of the administration can be checked by multiple individuals.

To help ensure that the drug is checked correctly a systematic approach can be used. A long-standing approach to this is often referred to as the 5Rs:

- Right patient
- Right drug
- Right time
- Right dose
- Right route.

Whilst these are helpful and essential things to check, they can provide a false sense of security if they are considered too superficially. These checks are intended to be more than simply confirming that the drug to be administered matches what has been prescribed; they are intended to make sure that the prescription itself is correct.

Right patient

Many care environments can have a large number of patients with a diverse range of conditions. It is essential that the patient is identified and their identity confirmed. The possibility that drug charts or directions to administer drugs could get confused cannot be ignored, even if the likelihood seems remote.

Checking the identity should usually involve the confirmation of multiple biographical details (e.g. name, date of birth, and address); if the patient has been provided with a hospital identification bracelet this can also be used to confirm identity. An identification bracelet can also be useful if the patient is unconscious or is otherwise unable to communicate.

Right drug

Checking that you are administering the correct drug is naturally an essential part of the checking process. However, identifying that the drug to be administered matches what has been prescribed is not the same as ensuring it is right for the patient.

Rapid Medicines Management for Healthcare Professionals, First Edition. Paul Deslandes, Simon Young and Ben Pitcher.
© 2020 John Wiley & Sons Ltd. Published 2020 by John Wiley & Sons Ltd.

Before administering a drug, a practitioner must be confident that use of the drug is in the patient's best interests and that it is compatible with any other therapy or treatment they are receiving. It is therefore necessary for the practitioner to consider the following points:

- Does the drug treat the condition the patient has? To answer this the practitioner should have some understanding of the nature and pathology of the patient's condition and the pharmacology of the drug prescribed.
- Does the patient have any conditions that would contraindicate the use of the drug to be administered? This may include long term co-morbidities (e.g. gastric ulcers contraindicate non-steroidal anti-inflammatory drugs) or acute changes in a patient's status that would make the drug unsafe to use (e.g. hypoglycaemia and insulin).
- Does the patient have an allergy to the drug? A patient's allergy status should be recorded on the patient's documentation and often on a bracelet. It is, however, also important to ask the patient to confirm that they have no allergy and be aware that an allergy may extend to all members of a group of drugs (e.g. allergy to penicillin means allergy to all members of that group, such as flucloxacillin, phenoxymethylpenicillin, or amoxicillin). Patients will not have identity bracelets in community settings and this means clear communication is paramount.

Right time

The timing of drug dosing can be important. Doses are typically equally spaced through the day to ensure that the drug plasma levels remain steady. Sometimes drugs are dosed at specific times to help minimise the impact of adverse effects or a specific period before or after meals. Administering drugs at the wrong time can impact upon their effectiveness, potentially causing gaps in therapy, and if they are given too close together can result in toxicity. Particular care should be taken if the drug is PRN (pro re nata) which means that the drug is given as required based upon the symptoms of the patient. It is important to check when the last dose was administered and if there is maximum amount of the drug that it is safe to administer over a given time period.

It is also important to be aware of the duration of the treatment. Whilst in some chronic conditions a drug may need to be administered for extended periods of time, acute conditions (such as infections) may require a course of medication for a finite period of time. Continuing the dosing of a medication beyond the intended period could negatively impact upon the patient.

Right dose

Even if the right drug has been confirmed, it must be used at the correct dose. If the drug dose is too high then it can be toxic, if is too low then it will be ineffective. When checking whether the dose is correct it is important to ensure you know for what indication the drug has been prescribed. For example, aspirin should usually be administered in doses of 600mg for pain but only 75mg when used as an antiplatelet.

Some drug doses must be calculated according to weight (or in rarer cases body surface area), and therefore an accurate and up-to-date body weight must be checked.

Dose adjustments may also be required to account for a patient's age or to account for other medical conditions or co-morbidities they may have. This can include low body weight or reduced renal or hepatic function.

The dosage of some drugs may also be adjusted according to specific patient measurements such as the dose of warfarin in line with international normalised ratio measurements and the dose of insulin in line with blood glucose monitoring.

Right route

The correct drug must be administered by the correct route. In many circumstances a drug may only available in one formulation, but some drugs can be supplied in multiple formulations and administered via different routes. For example, paracetamol is most commonly thought of as oral medication, but it can also be given intravenously. Ensuring that the drug is administered by the correct route is essential, as different routes may require different doses and have differing onsets of action.

It is also important to consider that the formulation of the drug is correct. A particular formulation may be required for the patient, for example a syrup or oral suspension may be required if the patient has swallowing difficulties.

Record keeping

When involved in any aspect of medicines administration it is essential for an accurate record of the administration to be kept. This is particularly important when a patient is in a hospital environment where the care may be undertaken by multiple individuals. If a proper record of administration has not been kept, additional doses of the same medicine may inadvertently be administered, resulting in an overdose and possible patient harm.

Within hospital environments, the most common means of recording the medications that have been administered is the drug chart. This paper document lists all the drugs a patient is to be given along with the doses, timings, and route. When a drug is administered the practitioner signs their initials (as does anyone who was involved in checking the medication) on the chart to denote that the drug has been administered and by whom.

The drug chart should also be annotated if the drug is not given. This may be due to the patient refusing the drug, being unable to take the drug or the drug being unavailable. As the space available to record this is usually limited on the chart, the information should also be recorded in the patient's notes.

Records should be contemporaneous (recorded as near to the event as possible) and should be recorded legibly in ink. Computerised record-keeping systems are becoming more prevalent in an effort to reduce reliance on paper-based systems, which can be damaged or lost.

Clinical note

The checking mechanisms discussed in this chapter are intended to detect errors and prevent them reaching the patient. If when undertaking these checks you identify an error, you should record it and report it via the appropriate mechanism employed in your area of practice.

81 Covert Administration

Administering medication to a patient without their knowledge is known as covert administration.

The Nursing and Midwifery Council state (with regards to covert administration):

> The registrant would need to be sure what they are doing is in the best interests of the patient, and that they are accountable for this decision.

If a patient has the mental capacity to make independent decisions about their treatment and their care, medication should not be given covertly. If, however, the patient lacks the capacity to make that decision and it is deemed in their best interest then medication can be administered covertly. When medication is administered in this way, it is often disguised and 'hidden' in food and or drink. All settings where covert administration may need to take place should have a process in place that follows contemporary laws and professional/regulatory guidelines. Guidelines are there to protect the patient but also protect those who are aware that covert administration is taking place. This often includes the patient's immediate family/guardians, the prescriber, the dispensing team, and those who are administrating the medication.

National Institute for Health and Care Excellence (NICE) suggest a process for managing and monitoring covert medication administration that is applied in care homes but has application in other settings where covert administration takes place. NICE suggest that any process that supports the administration of covert medication should consider:

- 'how to assess someone's capacity to refuse a medicine and how to record reasons for presuming a person's incapacity
- holding a meeting to determine what is best for the person
- recording the proposed treatment plan and the reason for giving a medicine without the person knowing
- planning how to give the medicine without the person knowing
- regularly reviewing whether covert administration is still needed'.

(NICE, 2014)

Considerations of giving medication covertly

If a patient lacks the mental capacity to make a decision with regard to taking a medication then a provider should consider the evidence needed to proceed with administering the medication covertly. The provider of the healthcare service may need to provide this evidence for consideration at a best interests meeting. The provider should provide evidence that they have a policy on administration of covert medication and that all of the relevant staff who may need to access that policy are able to do so. Staff will need to be appropriately trained in the legal considerations, e.g. they should have an appropriate understanding

Rapid Medicines Management for Healthcare Professionals, First Edition. Paul Deslandes, Simon Young and Ben Pitcher.
© 2020 John Wiley & Sons Ltd. Published 2020 by John Wiley & Sons Ltd.

of the relevant legislation and their training should cover issues around capacity and consent. Evidence concerning the themes of capacity, the role of the best interests meeting and its attendees, and patient care planning is also obtained before covert medication administration is undertaken.

Legal considerations: medicinal products

Changing medicines by, for example, crushing tablets to add to food or drink, or to pass down a percutaneous endoscopic tube is more often than not an off-label activity. This is a method of administration that the manufacturer of the product has not tested. Due to a lack of evidence suggesting this is a safe and efficacious way to use the medication it cannot be condoned by the manufacturer. Prescribing medicines in a manner outside of the recommendations of the marketing authorisation alters and increases the prescriber's professional responsibility and liability. Nurses who are not independent prescribers are not allowed to authorise the use of medicines outside of their marketing authorisation. Therefore, if medicines are to be administered covertly, this must be authorised by a relevant prescriber.

Pharmaceutical considerations

There is little detailed evidence regarding the stability of medicines when they are mixed with food or drink (except if the manufacturers have tested this before the medication comes to market). There is therefore a balance to be struck between putting a medication in food/drink and the effect on the medication's stability and the patient not receiving the medication.

In addition to the issues discussed above:

1. Medicines may become unacceptable to patients when hidden in food. Some medicines may have unpleasant and bitter tastes and may have a local anaesthetic effect in the mouth. This may result in the patient spitting out food (and the accompanying medication). This will result in a missed dose but may also have a detrimental effect on the ongoing acceptability of food. This in turn may have a deleterious effect on the patient if they are underweight or refusing food because of mental health impairment.
2. Pharmacokinetics also need to be considered – some medications need to be taken before food or on an empty stomach. The addition of food here will lead to suboptimal dosing.
3. Some medicines (e.g. the tetracyclines) interact with food and calcium-containing products such as dairy products.
4. Crushing medicine has implications for the person undertaking the administration. Cytotoxic drugs and some other medications that may be teratogenic may come into contact with the person undertaking the administration. This would not be the case if tablet were just "popped form blisters". Crushing slow or modified-release preparations is not recommended as the release characteristics of the drug from the formulation are changed and as a consequence the clinical effectiveness and expected response may not be as predicted.

Covert administration should be considered carefully and judged to be the correct clinical decision from all dimensions of care before it is undertaken.

Reference

NICE (2014) Managing medicines in care homes: When care home staff give medicines without a resident knowing. Social care guideline [SC1]. Available at https://www.nice.org.uk/guidance/sc1/ifp/chapter/When-care-home-staff-give-medicines-without-a-resident-knowing.

82 Evidence-based Medicine

What is evidence-based medicine?

Evidence-based medicine (EBM) aims to optimise the treatment that a patient receives through the use of research-based evidence rather than tradition or personal preference.

Using published literature to inform practice in this way forms the basis of EBM. In order to be published, papers must be submitted to journals and be peer-reviewed by other researchers working in the relevant field. The aim of peer-review is to help to ensure the quality of published papers. Whilst the majority of published findings have been peer-reviewed, the applicability of these studies to clinical practice cannot always be guaranteed. Most study designs are inherently limited in some way, and an awareness of some of these potential problems may be useful when assessing their relevance to practice.

Study design

It is often stated that the 'gold-standard' approach to assessing the efficacy of a treatment is the randomised controlled trial (RCT). Here, subjects are randomly assigned to a treatment or comparator, and differences in outcome between the two evaluated. These studies are designed to control factors (bias) that may influence the outcome, so that the true effect of the treatment can be estimated. In order to limit potential differences between individual subjects (and therefore possible bias), subjects are selected on the basis of strict inclusion and exclusion criteria. Subjects are allocated to treatment or comparator groups at random to minimise any differences between the groups. If the study is blinded, it means that either the researcher or the participant (single blinded) or both (double blinded) are unaware of the treatment they are receiving. This also helps to reduce potential bias.

These studies are useful when answering a specific question, but may not be very applicable (or generalisable) to day-to-day clinical practice. Many typical patients might be excluded due to the inclusion and exclusion criteria, and a short study duration (typically a period of a few weeks) may not be able to provide answers relating to the long-term use of the medicine under investigation. Studies using less strict criteria that are designed to be more representative of clinical practice (pragmatic studies) can overcome some of these limitations, but by their nature might be more susceptible to bias.

In some cases, an RCT or pragmatic study design may not be appropriate due to ethical considerations or the scale of the population to be studied. In such cases, so-called observational studies (e.g. cohort and case-control studies) can be applied. Here, a group of patients who have been treated with a given medicine might be identified (typically from a database) and their outcomes established. These studies are more susceptible to bias and cannot typically prove a causative link between the intervention and outcome. However, they can collect data on large numbers of patients, which might not otherwise be feasible in an RCT.

Rapid Medicines Management for Healthcare Professionals, First Edition. Paul Deslandes, Simon Young and Ben Pitcher.
© 2020 John Wiley & Sons Ltd. Published 2020 by John Wiley & Sons Ltd.

Statistical analysis and the *P* value

A key component of study reporting is statistical analysis. The nature of the analysis will vary with the study design. However, studies tend to be based on the idea that a small sample of patients with a given disorder is investigated and the results are used to make assumptions about everyone with that disorder. If a treatment makes a difference in the study sample, would that difference be found if you were able to investigate everyone with the disorder?

A common feature quoted for most statistical outcomes is the *P* value. The *P* value gives an indication of whether or not a difference between treatments in a study is statistically significant. The *P* value is a numerical value between one and zero. The smaller the *P* value, the less likely it is that there is no difference between the treatments. Statistical significance (suggesting that there is a difference between treatments in a study) is typically assumed when the *P* value for a given statistical test is less than 0.05 ($P < 0.05$).

It is important to note that a trial may be able to identify a *statistical difference* between treatments ($P < 0.05$), but this does not necessarily mean that there is a *clinically significant difference* between treatments. The interpretation of whether or not the study indicates a clinically significant difference is largely a matter for clinical judgment.

Reviewing literature

The quality of reporting of trial outcomes in published literature has often been criticised. It may be the case that the person or organisation conducting the trial has a vested interest in the outcome. A pharmaceutical company may wish to provide evidence in support of the use of their medicine, for example. There are a number of ways in which the publication of trial findings can be manipulated to meet the aims of the investigator. Selective reporting of positive study outcomes (and non-reporting of negative outcomes) may occur, whilst studies not showing the desired outcome may not be published at all. Furthermore, falsified results may be published and not identified unless a subsequent study fails to replicate the original findings.

When evaluating studies, a few key questions can help to determine the relevance to your practice. It is important to establish whether the study design is appropriate to investigate the desired outcome and whether the outcome is relevant to practice. Are the participants representative of those you see in practice and are there enough of them to investigate the study aim? Has ethical approval been sought and obtained where appropriate? Is the study appropriately blinded (where appropriate) or does the nature of the intervention limit the ability to blind the study? Have all of the subjects been accounted for in the analysis and have all the pre-stated outcomes been reported? Are conclusions based on the pre-stated primary outcome measure (the main outcome that the study was designed to investigate) or on other secondary outcome measures (which may not have been the intended focus of the study)?

Glossary

5-hydroxytryptamine (5-HT)   See serotonin.

Acetylcholine   A neurotransmitter in the central and peripheral nervous systems.

Activated partial thromboplastin time (aPTT)   A way of assessing blood clotting, commonly used for patients prescribed heparin.

Adrenaline (epinephrine)   A neurotransmitter and hormone in the central and peripheral (sympathetic) nervous systems.

Adverse drug reaction   An unwanted, harmful effect of a medicine.

Anaphylaxis   An acute, life-threatening, allergic reaction.

Ante cibum (ac)   Before food.

Appropriate polypharmacy   NICE defines appropriate polypharmacy as "Prescribing for a person for complex conditions or for multiple conditions in circumstances where medicines use has been optimised and where the medicines are prescribed according to best evidence."

Bioavailability   The proportion of an administered drug that reaches the bloodstream.

Biologic medicine   A complex medicine produced using a biotechnological process.

Biosimilar   A medicine that is similar but not identical to, and which is intended to be used for the same indication as an original biologic medicine.

British National Formulary (BNF)   A standard source of up-to-date information about medicines aimed at healthcare professionals.

Buccal   Part of the cheek and oral mucosa sometimes used as a route of administration.

Caution   A situation where extra care is needed when using a medicine.

Clinical Knowledge Summaries   An electronic resource available via the NICE evidence website, providing evidence-based advice relating to the management of a range of clinical conditions in primary care.

Concomitant   Use of two or more medicines together.

Contraindication   A situation where a medicine should not be used.

Controlled drug   A drug whose prescription, supply, and storage are subject to additional considerations due to the risk of misuse and harm.

Coumarins   A group of anticoagulant drugs that includes warfarin.

Cytochrome P450   A family of enzymes responsible for the metabolism of many drugs and other substances.

Dopamine   A neurotransmitter in the central and peripheral nervous systems.

Drug interaction   A change in the effect of a medicine resulting from its combined use with one or more other substances.

Electronic Medicines Compendium   A searchable, online repository of patient information leaflets (PIL) and summaries of product characteristics (SmPC).

Epinephrine   See adrenaline.

Estimated glomerular filtration rate (eGFR)   An estimation of renal function.

Excipient   A constituent of a drug formulation that is not the active ingredient.

Rapid Medicines Management for Healthcare Professionals, First Edition. Paul Deslandes, Simon Young and Ben Pitcher.
© 2020 John Wiley & Sons Ltd. Published 2020 by John Wiley & Sons Ltd.

Extra-pyramidal side effect (EPSE)   A group of movement disorders (e.g. pseudoparkinsonism) that are adverse effects of certain medicines that block dopamine neurotransmission, such as antipsychotics.

Formulation   The way in which a medicine is presented for administration (e.g. tablet, suppository, eyedrops).

Gamma-aminobutyric acid (GABA)   The principal inhibitory neurotransmitter in the central nervous system.

Glutamate   The principal excitatory neurotransmitter in the central nervous system.

Histamine   A chemical signalling molecule associated with allergy and gastric acid secretion.

Iatrogenic   An illness caused by medical treatment.

Idiopathic   A disorder of spontaneous or uncertain cause.

Inappropriate polypharmacy   NICE defines inappropriate polypharmacy as "The prescribing of multiple medicines inappropriately, or where the intended benefit of the medicines are not realised."

Indication   A condition or disorder for which a drug is used.

International normalised ratio (INR)   A way of assessing blood clotting, commonly used for patients prescribed warfarin.

International Unit   A unit of measurement based on biological activity (as opposed to mass or volume) and used as the dosing measure for certain drugs (e.g. insulin and certain vitamins).

Ligand   A molecule that binds to a receptor.

Marketing authorisation
(formerly Product Licence)   Permission from a regulator for a medicine to be marketed for specific use(s) in clinical practice.

National Institute for Health and Care Excellence (NICE)   A national body providing guidance, advice, and other information for healthcare professionals, and appraisal guidance on the cost-effectiveness of new medicines for use in England and Wales. The NICE Evidence website provides electronic access to the BNF and Clinical Knowledge Summaries for specific conditions.

Neuroleptic malignant syndrome   A potentially life-threatening adverse effect of antipsychotic drugs.

Neuron(e)   A nerve cell.

Neurotransmitter   A chemical signalling molecule that allows transmission of a message between neuron(e)s.

Noradrenaline (norepinephrine)   A neurotransmitter in the central and peripheral (sympathetic) nervous systems.

Norepinephrine   See noradrenaline.

Off-label   Use of a licensed medicine outside the conditions of its marketing authorisation.

Opiate   A drug based on the structure of opium alkaloids (e.g. morphine).

Opioid   A ligand acting through opioid receptors, resulting in similar actions to those of opium alkaloids.

Patient group direction (PGD)   A mechanism that allows supply of a medicine for a specific group of patients without the need for a prescription.

Peak flow   A way of assessing lung function.

Polypharmacy   See appropriate polypharmacy and see inappropriate polypharmacy

Post cibum (pc)   With or after food.

Prescription   An order allowing the legal supply of a medicine.

Pro re nata (PRN)   An instruction used to denote as required use of a medicine in response to symptoms.

Receptor   A protein molecule which, when bound to by an agonist ligand, can mediate a physiological response.

Serotonin (5-hydroxytryptamine, 5-HT)   A neurotransmitter in the central and peripheral nervous systems.

Side effects   Effects of a medicine that are separate from its main therapeutic effect. Side effects are typically caused by an action of the medicine at a site other than the one responsible for its therapeutic effect.

Stevens–Johnson syndrome   A rare but potentially fatal skin condition that may occur due to a hypersensitivity adverse reaction to a medicine.

Summary of Product Characteristics (SmPC)   A document produced by the manufacturer providing comprehensive information relating to the safe and effective use of a medicine.

Teratogenesis   Abnormal physiological development of the foetus.

Therapeutic drug monitoring (TDM)   Measurement of the level of a drug in the body, typically through blood sampling.

Unlicensed medicine   A medicine that does not have marketing authorisation in the country of its use.

Index

Rapid Medicines Management for Healthcare Professionals, First Edition. Paul Deslandes, Simon Young and Ben Pitcher.
© 2020 John Wiley & Sons Ltd. Published 2020 by John Wiley & Sons Ltd.